Zap the Fat

Zap the Fat

John French

Foreword by Henry Novack, M.D.
Cardiologist
Board Certified Specialist
Cardiovascular Diseases

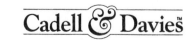

An imprint of Multi Media Communicators, Inc.
New York

Cadell & Davies™
An imprint of Multi Media Communicators, Inc.
575 Madison Avenue, Suite 1006
New York, NY 10022

Cadell & Davies™ is a trademark of Multi Media Communicators, Inc.

Library of Congress Cataloging-in-Publication Data

French, John P., 1930-
  Zap the fat/John P. French; foreword by Henry Novack.
    p. cm.
  ISBN: 1-56977-650-4

    1. Low-fat diet.   I. Title.

RM237.7.F74 1994
613.2'8—dc20   94-38778
                                                      CIP

10 9 8 7 6 5 4 3 2 1

Printed in the United States of America at Paraclete Press.

TO

BARRY

My wife...
  My editor...
    My Zap the Fat cook...
      My best friend.

ACKNOWLEDGMENTS

There are so many who have contributed to bringing *Zap the Fat* from a working program into a finished document. At the risk of failing to mention some, I must list a few.

Dr. David G. Wells, my personal physician since we moved to northern Arizona in 1991, who was the first to encourage me to create this detailed account of *Zap the Fat* for others to share.

Lillian Miao, my publisher, David Manuel, and Carol Showalter of 3D, for their relentless efforts to bring it all to fruition.

Joe Cox, Jr., for his Herculean work analyzing saturated fat figures on all food items and recipes.

Heart Smart Restaurants International, and its President, J. Philip French, Jr., for providing the data to analyze figures and check all the statistics regarding saturated fat.

Members of The Community of Living Water and The Community of Jesus for being guinea pigs, and for their ongoing work testing recipes for the desserts included in Appendix 1.

Dorothy Donnelly, Joannie Lautz, Hazel Meier, and Helen Waddoups, for developing dessert recipes that qualified for *Zap the Fat*, testing them, and proving to us how good they could taste.

Albert, Isabel, and Esther Kramer (and their Manzanita Inn), for demonstrating how a restaurant can adapt the *Zap the Fat* Program and still offer great tasting food.

Jay Shackelford, who got me started doing the weight lifting program explained in Chapter 9, and encouraged me to keep with it.

Dr. J. Matthew Roberts, for his valuable input regarding what it takes to break habit patterns.

TABLE OF CONTENTS

Foreword 1

Chapter 1 9
How It All Began

Chapter 2 19
How Does It Work?

Chapter 3 32
Changing the Habit Pattern

Chapter 4 39
Dairy and Eggs

Chapter 5 49
All About Meat

Chapter 6 61
Salad Dressings, Oils, and Margarine

Chapter 7 70
Breads, Desserts, and Candy

Chapter 8   80
    From Soup to Nuts (And Everything Else)

Chapter 9   88
    Making Exercise Simple

Chapter 10   97
    Easy Eating Out (Or, How To Convert
    Your Favorite Restaurant)

Chapter 11   107
    If Cholesterol and/or Sodium
    Are Your Problem

Chapter 12   119
    Postscript

Appendix 1   128
    Desserts That Make It All Worthwhile

Appendix 2   143
    Understanding Package Labels

***ZAP THE FAT*™ Wallet Card**   147

FOREWORD

Food is an essential part of our daily lives. We wake up thinking about it, plan our day around it, use it as a means to further business and to strengthen personal relationships. As a nation and individually, we are absorbed by food. Food is used as a reward, a punishment, a comfort, a stress-reliever, even a companion. For all these reasons and more, we eat whenever we feel like it rather than when we're hungry.

If we ate only when we were hungry, we'd eat a moderate amount perhaps every four to six hours. If we ate only when we were hungry, food would taste better—not so much stronger as deeper, richer, fuller. If we ate only when we were hungry, food would smell better—the aroma would fill our nostrils. If we ate only when we were hungry, food would feel more appealing to the tongue—delicate flakes of fish have a different sensate quality than robust hard rolls. If we ate only when we were hungry, food would be more gratifying for all our senses.

But because we eat for so many reasons unrelated to hunger, food doesn't satisfy. We eat a power breakfast—power in this case meaning one filled with business conversation rather than one power-packed with nutrition. We say we skip lunch because we're too busy, but in reality, we've been unconsciously snacking all morning. And rather than being television's idealized family time, dinner all too often is a lonely time to be avoided (which means fast food or pizza in front of the television), stress-filled with squalling kids and/or an angry spouse, shallow conversation with associates, or intense discussions with client or boss.

However, rather than any of the above, food's primary purpose is to provide the fuel to keep a person's machinery in good running order. (That's not a bad pun.) When food is used for other than its primary purpose, excess pounds ensue and the machinery runs amok. That's what we see happening today.

Coronary artery disease, diabetes, arthritis, lung cancer, breast cancer and a staggering number of other illnesses are affected by—and in many cases result from—excess poundage. I am a cardiologist. I see this every day. Obesity exacts an astounding toll on our lives.

Coronary artery disease remains the major cause of death among Americans. About 30 percent of the total U.S. population—perhaps 68 million people—suffer from some form of cardiovascular disease. And it is probable that more than 7 million adults are on their way to a heart attack. For the most part, this is due to their food habits. Coronary artery disease has been called the black plague of the affluent. The World Health Organization reports that 55 out of every 100,000 Americans die of coronary disease each year. In Switzerland, it's 33 for every 100,000 and in Japan, 15 per 100,000.

Excess poundage is the causative factor behind many modern scourges—not just coronary artery disease. An estimated 46,000 people will die this year from breast cancer. Researchers for several years have linked obesity to breast cancer and a recent study done in Tampa,

Florida, indicates the severity of the problem. Women who carry 10 extra pounds increase their risk of breast cancer by 23 percent; 15 pounds, 37 percent; 20 pounds, 52 percent.

Lung cancer now is the leading cause of death for women, and not just women who smoke. Researchers at the National Cancer Institute determined in a recent study that women with diets high in saturated fat—such as meat, butter and cheese—had about four times the usual risk of lung cancer, whether or not they smoked. More than 170,000 new cases of lung cancer will be diagnosed this year and 149,000 of them will die from it.

A recent article in the Journal of the American Medical Association reported on a 1991 survey by ethnicity that showed 33 percent of all Americans were overweight, and overweight was defined as 20 to 24 percent above ideal weight. That's about 25 pounds for a 5-foot-4-inch woman and 30 pounds for a 5-foot-10-inch man. Even worse, in virtually every age and race and in both sexes, the prevalence of obesity was higher than in the survey taken 30 years earlier—and in every instance, the prevalence climbed most dramatically in the last decade.

People do talk about the problem of excess poundage but apparently dieting isn't the answer. The June 1993 issue of *Consumer Reports* described its poll of 95,000 subscribers who tried to lose weight within the last three years. Almost 20,000 of the subscribers had gone to one of the five best-known weight-loss programs—Jenny Craig International, Nutri-System, Physician's Weight Loss Centers and Weight Watchers—or to one of three medically supervised liquid fasts. The average dieter regained almost half the weight lost within six months, and two-thirds of it within two years.

None of the five programs, all of which combine dieting and counseling, fared better than the others, *Consumer Reports* noted.

Overweight is a medical situation that brings with it
a host of other life-threatening problems, but apparently dieting isn't the answer. It doesn't solve the problem. Author John French is very careful—and emphatic—
in saying the information in his new book *Zap the Fat* is
not a diet. It's a life-style. It's a style of eating for life.

The life of a human being is irreplaceable. I believe
very strongly that all of us are unique; that no one can
ever be exactly like another person. And I believe very
strongly that we all were created for a purpose—not so
much for accomplishment of a task, but for each other.
Ultimately it is selfishness, then, that leads to death from
causes related to overweight. Do you think that is a harsh
statement? Think of what you say about food: "This is
something I do for myself." "This one's for me." "This
is my favorite." I, me, my. Selfishness.

And death from causes related to being overweight
isn't the only loss. There is a financial toll. In a recent
report released by the American Medical Association,
coronary heart disease costs Americans $49 billion an-
nually, directly and indirectly; strokes, $11 billion; and
diabetes, $13.8 billion. Obesity is just an extremely costly
problem.

Modification of identifiable risk factors helps lower
the threat of coronary disease. Diet, hypertension, ciga-
rette smoking and exercise all are areas that people
should look at before they become victims of coronary
disease. I find that one of the most difficult aspects of
the treatment of coronary disease is the dietary therapy.
It is difficult to explain to a patient the specifics of keeping a low fat intake. Even when using charts of cholesterol and fat content, it is difficult to plan. Dieticians

are helpful but I have been singularly unsuccessful in convincing patients to see them. Spotty coverage by many insurance plans is also a factor in patient failure to get a handle on how to eat therapeutically. This is to me the beauty of *Zap the Fat*. In an eminently readable fashion this book gives practical suggestions about how to maintain a fairly stringent low fat intake.

I am recommending *Zap the Fat* to all my patients. John French has developed a virtually painless way for people to control the amount of saturated fat in their diet, without sacrificing good taste and quality of life, and he provides in the book a convenient wallet-sized card to help people remember what they can safely— and tastefully—eat. *Zap the Fat* makes healthy eating understandable. That's the bottom line. *Zap the Fat* is understandable for the layperson.

Therapeutic eating apparently is one of the areas of life that people don't like to think about, because there is nothing imminently difficult about nutrition. Perhaps it is all just a bit overwhelming because of the sheer variety of the food that is available to us. In some developing countries, there is one staple, one main food item—oftentimes, that staple is rice. In the United States, on the other hand, there are many staples—and they vary by region. Not everyone eats a bagel for breakfast, but just try telling New Yorkers that! Its very name tells people where Southern fried chicken comes from, but it is a staple nationwide. Mexican food—rice, beans, frijoles—is another collective staple whose popularity has spread far from its origins. As a nation, we are far more pleasure-bound than perhaps is good for us, products of the television-induced immediate gratification syndrome that spawned too many of us. We don't want to have to think about what we're eating, and we don't want to give up eating anything that gives us pleasure.

Small wonder we're overweight!

But food improperly used shortens lives. How many seriously overweight people do you know who are more than 60 years old? Medical researchers have found that if you are 10 percent overweight, you have a 15 percent smaller chance of surviving the next 20 years; if you are 20 percent overweight, your chances are 25 percent less; if you are 30 percent overweight, 45 percent less.

Medical studies have shown that it is not how much a person eats but what they eat that adds unnecessary pounds. The main culprit, of course, is fat. Fat is a chemically complex food component that plays an essential role in the metabolic process: Fats provide more than twice the number of calories than do proteins and carbohydrates; they can be stored in the body in large quantities for later use; and they serve as carriers of fat-soluble vitamins A, D, E and K.

There are two kinds of fats, based on the differences in their molecular structure. If the carbon atoms in fat molecules are boxed in by hydrogen atoms, they are said to be saturated, densely packed together. This is what gives these fats their solid texture at room temperature. The carbon atoms in unsaturated fats are said to be free-floating because they are not boxed in by their smaller amounts of hydrogen atoms. They are, therefore, liquid at room temperature.

Saturated fats may liquefy at high temperatures, but they revert to their solid state—inside or outside your body—at room temperature.

Cholesterol is a separate entity altogether. Cholesterol is a fatty crystalline alcohol manufactured in a person's liver—about 2,000 milligrams a day—and necessary for almost every tissue in the body, such as some brain tissue and spinal tissue, which have cholesterol as one of their main structural components. In other words, like saturated fat, cholesterol has mass, bulk. It is not a liquid.

In addition to the naturally manufactured cholesterol—which is most of the amount your body needs—the average American adult ingests another 450 milligrams, depending on what food they eat, much of which collects (for reasons we're still not sure about) in the two pencil-thin arteries that take blood away from the heart. As the cholesterol collection grows, less and less blood is able to leave the heart and do its proper work in the heart muscle cells. A fullblown heart attack happens when bloodstarved heart tissue dies.

Cholesterol is related to saturated fat because food high in saturated fat contributes to a high cholesterol level. This is why the medical community is telling people with high cholesterol levels to decrease the amount of saturated fat in their diets. Several studies have shown that a significant change in eating habits—specifically, cutting down on saturated fat—results in an almost immediate decrease in the cholesterol level and an increase in the ability of blood to flow freely from the heart.

One recent study combined the results of 22 trials involving more than 40,000 subjects. In the 14 trials conducted for less than four years, a 10 percent reduction in serum cholesterol led to a 10 percent reduction in coronary events. The eight trials conducted for longer periods of time showed a doubling of this benefit, leading to 20 percent fewer coronary events. The Oslo trial, which also included smoking cessation, showed a 13 percent reduction in total cholesterol over five years, compared to 3 percent in the control group. The combination in this small trial led to a 47 percent reduction in heart attacks and sudden death, and 53 percent reduction in death from coronary disease.

Zap the Fat is a book that gives information in concise, everyday language that wise people will use to adjust their daily food habits to benefit their health all the way around. As John French says, this is not a diet; it's a life-style—a life-style you can live with.

This book is what I'm giving my patients to help them understand the basics of good nutrition, therapeutic eating that does not shorten life. I especially like the emphasis on exercise as well. While the intensity the author recommends does not have to be followed exactly, even 20 minutes of brisk walking 3-4 times a week has been shown to have benefit. Because *Zap the Fat* provides a way of easily controlling fat intake, it has solved a problem for my patients—and, I hope, for you.

Henry F. Novack, M.D. FACC, *professor at Columbia Presbyterian School of Medicine, in clinical practice at St. Luke's Roosevelt Hospital Center, New York City.*

1

HOW IT ALL BEGAN

It was June of 1986. I was 56 years old. My wife, Barry, and I were touring England with her aunt and our granddaughter. That meant driving on the left side of the road. I didn't handle that well.

In fact, there were many times I hardly handled it at all. I had a tendency to get too far to the left and contacted some curbs abruptly. Barry and I were always trying to get in the door on the wrong side of the car.

Then there were those prickly English hedgerows that grow right up to and over onto the roads. And the ditches. Each with a precipitous drop-off. Wherever there wasn't a hedgerow I found a ditch. It seemed that I was running our small Ford into one or the other most of the first few days.

But where it really got to me was the right turns. Somehow swinging out to turn and maneuvering at once to the left side of the road really stressed me out.

Then there were those charming old inns. We had chosen them to add to the atmosphere of the trip. Of course, we ended up on the third (and one time fourth) floor of every one of them.

With my three women companions, there were a lot of bags to carry up and down all those flights of stairs.

Still, it all seemed to be going fine. Until we arrived

in London. We were spending the last four days of our trip there at another charming, small, old hotel.

The first night it hit me. A sharp pain in my chest. It seemed the same as some muscular pains I had suffered in years past. But the next morning, this one hadn't gone away as had always been the case in the past.

I was sure the strain of staying out of the hedgerows and the ditches while driving on the left side of the road plus carrying all those bags was the culprit. My chest muscles were surely crying out in rebellion.

I got through the next day by hanging on to my self-deception. Even another sleepless night. But the next morning Barry decided she had had enough of this foolishness. She called for the house doctor.

They didn't have one. However, they did line up an appointment for us to go see a man who claimed that title in his "surgery."

After a jostling cab ride we arrived at his so-called surgery. It was a scene right out of a World War I movie. Straight chairs. Porcelain covered counters. Medieval looking instruments arranged on large trays. A yellowish-tan painted wall that was anything but comforting. And the doctor. He, too, fit the scene perfectly. White hair. Very proper. No receptionist. No nurse. No assistant. No names on doors.

No confidence!

Listening to my heart, the doctor agreed that it must be a matter of muscles. He gave me a prescription for what he identified as a muscle relaxant and sent me to the pharmacy at the hospital in the next block. There we were handed one of those old-fashioned glass bottles with a screw top and an ample supply of muscle relaxant.

It was all for nought. After another sleepless night we flew back to the States. The pain continued until the night I got back in my own bed in Phoenix. Then miraculously, it went away. Still, since I had told my doctor at that time about the problem, he insisted I come in to let him check me out.

A stress test revealed no serious problem. Just some minor irregularities. So a few weeks later we were on our way to our summer home in Michigan.

For some years I had spent 10 minutes a day jumping on a small trampoline. I didn't know it at the time but that was what had saved my life.

Since we spent a couple of months in Michigan each summer I also kept a trampoline there. The day we arrived, I climbed on it for the first time since we had returned from England. That lasted less than 30 seconds.

Something like a knot hit me in the chest the moment my heart beat increased. The same thing happened when I went up a small incline on the walk to our house. And again when I got out on the golf course. Always from just slight inclines. What was the matter?

My doctor in Phoenix exploded with an expletive when I called him to report this latest series of events. He sent me 100 miles away to Grand Rapids to run a another stress test. It showed no change so he felt that if I did not exert myself, it was OK to wait until I got back in September to run more tests and find out what was in there.

Before returning to Phoenix, we were scheduled to attend a conference in West Virginia. About a week before our scheduled departure we were guests at a dinner party at our next door neighbor's home.

It was a lovely night. The company was interesting. The food was heavy, delicious, and loaded with fat (at this point I still paid no attention to what I ate because I had no idea what really was bad for me). The only problem was that it was past nine o'clock before they got around to serving. I nibbled for more than an hour before dinner, and then overate.

Right after dinner I was exhausted. We started the short walk to our house next door, a distance of about 200 feet.

On the way I was forced to stop three times to get my breath. And rest. By the time we reached the front door Barry exclaimed, "If you think I am going to fly to D.C. and drive five hours down into the mountains of West Virginia with you in this condition, you have really lost it."

So we went directly home to Phoenix. The day after we arrived, my cardiologist set a date two days later for me to go into the hospital for an angiogram. He seemed confident it wasn't any problem we couldn't handle easily with a few drugs.

The morning of the angiogram Barry drove me to the hospital. I was scared. I had heard what was in store for me from friends who had had the same procedure.

After an attendant had shaved and prepped my lower torso, I concluded it was time to just settle in for what promised to be a long list of new experiences. Some frightening. Some embarrassing. Some downright humiliating.

When we got into the operating room they loaded me with enough drugs to keep me drowsy but still awake. The doctor had explained it was necessary to keep me awake during the procedure.

His first step was to make an incision in the artery in my groin. That was painless. Then (still without any pain) he inserted a tube with a light on the end into that artery. He let it wind its way up into my heart.

"Look," the doctor said, staring into my clouded eyes.

"You can see where you created your own bypass. That was probably the cause of the pain you experienced in England."

I gave one furtive glance, enough to realize I did not want to see any more. I had absolutely no desire to look at the inside of my heart. Or anything else inside of me. I had never done well around blood and this was certainly no exception.

After that first look, the doctor inserted a dye into the tube. More excitement. Within minutes I was breaking out with hives all over my body. They had to inject another drug to counteract the hives. I was sure this whole event was about all I could take of hospitals and doctors and operating rooms for a long time to come.

A few hours after the procedure, the doctor came into my hospital room where Barry and I were chatting. When he pulled a chair up to the bed, I sensed that the solution to my problem was not going to be as simple as we had hoped. I was beginning to realize that not only was I not liking where I was, but I also was not going to like what I was about to hear.

"One artery is 70% blocked, but the big problem is the main one, which is 100% blocked," he said gently.

He explained how I had created my own bypass. The veins that went around the blockage were carrying enough blood to keep me from having an outright heart attack. The pain came whenever I exerted any effort, because I was then forced to pump more blood through this narrow opening than it could handle.

The good news was that my years of daily workouts on the trampoline had paid off. I had created sufficient optional paths for the blood to flow through that I had not had a heart attack when the artery closed entirely. Indeed, the doctor and his team had all been astounded to see that I was still walking around.

He explained that the location of the blockages ruled out the new balloon method they were using to open clogged arteries. My only option was heart bypass surgery. The sooner the better.

My thoughts immediately went to several of my friends living at The Community of Jesus on Cape Cod who had had this same operation at Massachusetts General Hospital in Boston.

They all had the same cardiologist and the same surgeon. Most important, they all had come through with flying colors and were now quite healthy. I knew Massachusetts General had an entire floor regularly filled with dozens of patients recovering from heart surgery. It sounded like the place to be.

I was 20 pounds over my proper weight at the time. That may not seem like much to you, but it was too much for my 5 foot 10 inches of very small bones.

(I am purposely not giving my exact weight throughout this book. The purpose of *Zap the Fat* is to allow our bodies to find the right weight for each of us individually and to stay there. Consequently, I deliberately avoid mentioning any weight that someone could erroneously try to use as a bench mark.)

My pants were too tight. I recently had to have all of them let out. I had never been able to stand clothing that fit tightly. The first time I took my teen-age daughters to a hockey game they had exclaimed, "Look, Dad, those hockey shorts are baggies, just like your pants!"

In fact, it had taken years of wrong eating to get me up there, some 40 pounds heavier than I was when I graduated from college.

A month after the angiogram I entered Mass General. It was quite a production. For a full day before the operation, they poked and probed every vein and body crevice. Barry joined me at several preparation sessions where they explained what was going to happen and how it would change my life forever.

By the time I finally went to surgery the next morning I was well drugged. Still I remember watching the lights go by as they rolled me to the operating room. My only thought was that this was not an experience I would like to repeat.

The operation seemed to go fine. It lasted for six hours. When Barry first visited me in the Recovery Room the next morning she said I was still ice cold with a unique gray color. After all, they had been running my blood through a machine outside my body all during the operation, and had to drop my body temperature down below 80 degrees.

I was out of it and really had little idea what was going on. But by the time they took me to my room the afternoon of the day following the operation, things seemed to look good.

My friends had all been in the hospital a week or less after their operations. The day after I was taken from recovery to my room they had me up and walking. I felt better than I had in years because the blood was flowing. I even had color in my face. That got the juices flowing.

I had always been what is termed a classic Type A personality. I would always try to do at least two things at a time. I regularly read a paper while I was talking on the phone.

I was also great at finishing other people's sentences. A leisurely walk was never part of my vocabulary.

I still detest having to wait in any line. If ever forced to do so, I make certain I have something along to read. I also like to count how many people are ahead of me. Then I observe just how long it is taking to serve each one. That way I can determine the amount of time it should take me to get to the head of the line.

I also can be tormented until I get something finished. Everything is measured in my mind by how far it is from completion. It's as if I breathe a sigh of relief when I finish any project.

I am inclined to make a numbers game out of almost anything. If I don't take control of myself I will time what I am doing to see if I'm doing it faster this time than the last. It's really sick!

A good friend of mine said once, "Johnny, you really are a sad case. You are so busy looking for the conclusion of everything that you miss all the fun finding out what's going to happen along the way to getting there."

This hospital stay was no exception. I was determined to get out in the least possible time. By the third day I was attending what was supposed to be my first and last discharge class.

It was in this class that a dietician tried to educate patients on the life-changing diet we were facing. The culprits we had to learn all about and watch for were cholesterol and fat. The diet was very involved—cholesterol seemed pretty easy, but how was I ever going to keep up with all that fat business?

No more than 30% of what I ate was to be fat—but 30% of what? Or, stated another way, limit yourself to 50 grams of fat a day—but that meant carrying around a good-sized book with tables needed to figure it all out.

A few days later I developed complications that kept me in the hospital exactly five weeks. So much for Type A John. But this also meant that I kept attending those discharge classes, several times a week, since they never knew when I would be well enough to be discharged.

I got to know the diminutive Korean dietician quite

well. I enjoyed trying to trip her up on the impossibility of carrying out all she was telling me—being a good Type A, it never occurred to me that no normal person could really learn to function with it all. Sometimes she acknowledged the intangibility of the whole thing—other times she grew quite adamant.

But even with my plethora of discharge classes, it was all still terribly confusing. There was hydrogenated fat, polyunsaturated fat, monosaturated fat, saturated fat, partially hydrogenated fat, good fat and bad fat. And a certain percentage of each that you were supposed to have each day.

Barry picked up a number of low-fat cookbooks at the hospital gift shop that we poured over. The more we read, however, the greater the problem seemed to become.

Even with my Type A love of dealing with detail, it was hopelessly confusing. How could anyone be expected to figure it out? How then could anyone hope to avoid being one of the 50% of those in each discharge class who the doctors predicted would be back within 10 years to have another heart bypass operation?

Still, Barry and I both struggled. My father, both of my grandfathers, and one of my grandmothers had debilitating strokes while still in their 60s, my father when he was just 61.

My cholesterol had been 350 prior to the operation. Both of my brothers also have naturally high cholesterol. The dietician had persuaded me that fat in the diet was the big problem, but how to cope with it in the midst of this maze of data?

The struggle went on for more than a year. My weight had dropped by 20 pounds during my hospital stay. The doctor put me on a cholesterol-lowering drug (Mevacor), and I spent a great deal of my time pouring over all those fat charts. As a result, my cholesterol stayed in the range of 220-230. Not the greatest, but apparently the best I could hope to do. (As I have continued on *Zap the Fat*, it has dropped to just over 200.)

But my weight was another problem. It had sneaked back up 10 pounds. I can always tell when I have too much weight because it goes to my face and my waist (those tight pants, again). Actually, this excess weight was also a signal that I was not doing all that should be done to lower the cholesterol, but I wasn't aware of that yet.

2

HOW DOES IT WORK?

I continued to struggle, trying to comprehend and interpret the myriad types of fats and other no-no's I had learned about at all those discharge classes at Massachusetts General Hospital. It wasn't working.

About this time, my son, Philip, left his job with a national food chain in North Carolina and returned to Arizona to open his own restaurant.

It was great! Fine food. Delightful Arizona outdoor eating. Quite popular.

I remember the day it opened. We had gone for breakfast with a close friend. The hostess at the front desk greeted us with a wide smile. She seemed to really be glad we were there. The waitress was also pleasant to be around.

But instead of relaxing and enjoying the atmosphere along with the excellent food that was to come, my roving eye picked up on a "temporary opening" sign over the door that was crooked. My friend commented, "If ever I have a production job to be done, I would want to use your company. But when it comes to eating in a restaurant, I want it to be one Philip is running."

Since we often had been with him for lunch or dinner, Philip was aware of my problem in picking food items that wouldn't guarantee a return trip to the hospital for a repeat operation.

At first he did what so many other restaurants across the country were doing—put a little heart beside each item on the menu that seemed to be healthy, and referred casually to the American Heart Association and its guidelines at the bottom of the menu.

That lasted for about a month—as long as it took for the American Heart Association to learn about it and ask him to please stop referring to them at all.

In the meantime, I also had pointed out to Philip that some of the items he identified as being heart healthy really didn't meet the guidelines we had learned about at Mass General discharge classes. Since he was my son, he responded with more attention than you could expect from the average restaurateur who is too busy worrying about the line cook who just quit and what to do about the station of his best waitress who called in sick this morning.

After tedious hours spent studying the fat content and related data about the ingredients, he finally came up with several items for his menu that truly met those standards of 10% or less of calories from saturated fat, 30% or less from total fat, no more than 150 milligrams of cholesterol, and no more than 1100 milligrams of salt.

This took a lot of in-depth research and development. Almost all the recipes that finally qualified needed some type of alteration. Add just one tablespoon of olive oil instead of two to saute the vegetables. Use skim instead of 2% or whole milk in the cup custard. Use an egg substitute or egg whites in place of whole eggs to make the French toast.

It was extremely time-consuming and not the sort of thing your average restaurant owner or chef exactly embraces. Nor was it something my wife found particularly easy or enjoyable while trying to cook at home.

Philip and his chef really struggled to reach exactly the right combination of low-fat and low saturated fat, and good taste. This required finding the right quantity of substitutes that gave a dish the same taste and feel as if you had actually included the fat. But to the needy diner like myself, it was well worth the effort.

Once they mastered the recipes, they then needed to decide how to identify them on the menu. Obviously, the simple heart was out. But to take its place Philip came up with an eye-catching idea: a heart and the word "Dad" written on a line.

Then, at the bottom of the menu he placed the legend: "Items marked with 𝒟𝒶𝒹 meet heart healthy guidelines so that my Dad, who has had heart bypass surgery, can eat them."

It was quite a hit with the customers. More important, it brought in a lot of new business from customers who were concerned with healthy eating when they dined out.

The primary key to the success of each of these healthy menu items, however, was their taste. They had to taste at least as good as anything that they had replaced on the menu.

The customer was not asked to sacrifice the pleasant experience of an exciting meal when eating out in order to get one that met healthy guidelines.

But the problems, confusion, and stress Philip had gone through to arrive at this point reinforced in my mind the fact that no individual was ever going to figure it all out. There was no way I, or anyone who wasn't ready to spend hours a day on the subject, could determine the right quantity of the right kind of fat to consume every day.

Then, one particular thing about all those different

types of fat struck me. Despite other changes of opinion by the experts over the years, I had consistently heard and read without exception that the real culprit in our diet is *saturated fat.*

Saturated fat is solid at room temperature. It is found in all products of animal origin (e.g. meat and dairy products), plus nuts, oils, and two fruits. In food it is always a percentage of the total fat—can be as little as 10% or as much as almost 90%.

Non-saturated fat can also be made similar to saturated by a process called hydrogenation. Liquid oils are hydrogenated to make such things as vegetable shortening and stick margarine. This is why they are higher in saturated fat than the oils in their liquid form. By making them hydrogenated, manufacturers also prolong their shelf life.

I'd heard saturated fat described as a primary cause of heart disease like mine. Of many types of cancer. Of just bad health in general. Indeed, everywhere I turned, saturated fat, along with smoking, kept looming its ugly head as the primary thing to avoid for good health.

So I asked myself: could saturated fat also be the culprit that causes excessive weight? I decided to pursue an in-depth study of that question.

I began by analyzing the statistics comparing the saturated fat in different foods to the total of all types of fat in each one. I was amazed at the results.

In some foods (such as coconut oil), I discovered that almost 90% of the fat was saturated. In others (such as whole milk dairy products) fat runs to over 60% saturated. Yet in others (such as canola oil and safflower oil) saturated fat makes up under 10% of the total fat.

So, if saturated fat were the culprit causing weight problems as well as health problems in general, looking at total fat wasn't necessary to get the job done. And looking at total fat was so complicated it wasn't ever likely to get it done.

In fact, I was horrified to find how high the amount of saturated fat was in some of things that I had been eating regularly. Even though I was staying within my prescribed limits of total fat. Small wonder I was still gaining weight.

I had been motivated by a study done by the Harvard School of Public Health. It determined that the thinner a man is, the longer he is likely to live.

In fact, it showed that many can significantly extend their life spans by getting down to a weight that most tables would show as being downright skinny. That was certainly my experience.

For example, they showed that a 5 foot 10 inch man wanting to live as long as possible should weigh no more than 157 pounds. This is a full 31 pounds less than the upper USDA figure for that height, and 20% less than the average American man that size would be expected to weigh.

Further, the study showed that men in the thinnest fifth of the population were 60% less likely to die from heart disease than those who are heavier.

I was sold on the need to weigh less and was excited that I had found the method. I started concentrating only on the saturated fat in what I was eating. That was the beginning of what eventually I named the *Zap the Fat* eating program.

Originally, my interest was entirely aimed at avoiding more artery blockage and the resulting heart problem or stroke. A limit on saturated fat intake certainly made sense for that. In fact, it made more sense than worrying about all the other types of fat.

That was more than five years ago. The decision I made was quite simple: I would eat no more than 10 grams of saturated fat every day. That was way below the maximum allowed in different programs, yet was quite workable.

With this decision, I was delighted to discover that I no longer needed vast tables with pages of data. Instead, it was a system I could quickly and easily learn.

Since we traveled a lot and therefore frequently ate out, I was delighted that it proved as helpful and effective when ordering from a restaurant menu as when eating at home. Yet it was as simple as learning the multiplication tables, and equally applicable in all situations.

It worked for keeping the cholesterol levels acceptable. Mine stabilized in the 220 range. But that was just the beginning. The amazing by-product has been my weight.

Within weeks of starting to follow this one simple precept of 10 grams or less of saturated fat a day, with no other restrictions on quantity or type of food I ate, my weight dropped back to its normal level and has stayed there ever since. It really did zap the fat.

One of my great loves has always been cheese. I love it. In any form. Even as a child during the depression, one of my most rewarding Christmas gifts was always a tray of cheese for my very own—everything from Gouda to Limburger. I was sure I just couldn't live without cheese.

When I first was told to watch my cholesterol I was delighted to discover that a slice (1 ounce) of American cheese (and almost any other type) contained only about 25 milligrams of cholesterol. If I must limit myself to 300 milligrams of cholesterol a day, and wanted to eat it all up in cheese, I could consume 12 ounces of the stuff— a full 3/4 of a pound. What a deal.

Then I learned it wasn't just the cholesterol that I had to watch, but that I must start limiting my fat intake to about 50 grams per day. At first I was worried. But since American cheese has just 9 grams of total fat in a 1-ounce slice, this meant that I could have almost six 1-ounce slices in a day and still stay within that 50 gram total.

But then I learned about saturated fat! My eyes were opened wide. Out of that 9 grams of fat, two-thirds, or 6 grams, are saturated fat!

With a limit of 10 grams of saturated fat per day, this meant I would consume more than half a day's allotment eating just a single, one-ounce slice of cheese. That doesn't leave much room for anything else.

By comparison, a half ounce of peanuts (a normal sized serving) contains 7 grams of total fat, close to the 9 grams in that single ounce of cheese. But less than one of those grams is saturated fat. That's just 14% of the total fat in peanuts that is saturated.

This means that I could eat 10 servings of peanuts and still be under 10 grams of saturated fat. Yet if I was looking at total fat, with 50 grams per day allotted, that would equal only 7 servings of peanuts.

This was beginning to make sense.

Better still, I discovered there are really very few things that contain saturated fat. All dairy products (except total non-fat ones). Regular oils and dressings. Meats (though many are so low that they can be used regularly to make up the daily 10 gram allotment). Commercially baked goods (except bread and rolls which are fine). Soups and nuts. That's about it.

All fruits except for two have no saturated fat. All vegetables contain none. All non-fat dairy products (and the market is loaded with good tasting ones today) are okay. Cocoa, salsas, ketchup, mustard, and many other things which help dishes to taste good—all okay.

I was beginning to get excited. First, because I now

knew that it was no longer necessary to continue trying to do the impossible. For the first time I was dealing with something I found I could really get a handle on. Saturated fat!

Second, because I was now convinced that limiting myself to 10 grams of saturated fat a day was the right thing to do for my whole cardiovascular system.

Those 10 grams of saturated fat a day in an average diet of 1,800 calories make up 5% of the calories. The American Heart Association guidelines limit daily saturated fat consumption to 10% of calories consumed. That's twice as much as what you'll get with the *Zap the Fat* program. That's why *Zap the Fat* brings you to your proper weight and keeps you there.

Third, and most important to me, was the simplicity and lack of stress that this brought into my life. No more big books with tables to pour over. No more different types of fats to be concerned with. No more confusion.

Instead, I am able to deal with something so simple to identify and count that it all fits on a small, wallet-sized card that I carry with me at all times.

Once I had gathered it all together, knowledge about the saturated fat in items I couldn't eat was easy to memorize. It has remained an easy part of my daily life ever since.

Obviously, all of this originally came to pass for me because of my heart problem. It was a matter of life or death, so I was rather well motivated. And excess weight is certainly a similar motivation.

It makes no difference how much I eat in a day, my weight doesn't fluctuate by more than three pounds. Even when a heavy salt intake on a given day causes such a fluctuation, I still return to my proper weight within the next couple of days.

What I eat covers the waterfront. Wonderful desserts,

including chocolate ones made with cocoa, since it contains almost no saturated fat. All the bread I want whenever I want it. A glass or two of wine a day when I feel like it.

Large breakfast. Good lunches. Delicious dinners. Yet as long as the day's intake contains no more than 10 grams of saturated fat, my weight stays right there where it should be.

I remember having lunch one day with a rabbi friend of mine. We had been discussing the *Zap the Fat* program—the fact that all you needed to count was the saturated fat.

"You mean to tell me I can eat all of this tuna fish (it was a whole can). Slathered with this mayonnaise (Nalley's, it contained no saturated fat). Then pile it high on a couple of pieces of bread. Highlight it with some lettuce, tomato, and onion slices. And it won't affect my weight at all? But if I were to add a little schmear of butter it would have a disastrous effect on my weight? Incredulous!"

He just couldn't believe it. Can you? Will it work for you as it has for me?

My experience indicates it will when we are willing to make one decision. That decision is simple: to eat no more than a limit of 10 grams of saturated fat per day. And to decide to eat this way for life.

This is not a temporary diet. Rather, for the rest of our lives we need to decide to limit ourselves to 10 grams of saturated fat every day. (Sure, we can go over one day and under the next, but it must still average out to 10 grams per day.)

If we don't make that decision, we are wasting our time. We'll have to be satisfied with the ongoing roller coaster battle of the bulge. It's our decision. But it must be made. No decision *is* a decision.

Over the past several years I have had numerous friends who began following *Zap the Fat*. They have all experienced weight loss in varying degrees. About one in five has chosen to adopt *Zap the Fat* as a new way of life.

One of these was George. He lives close by and often has lunch with me, occasionally dinner. He started on the program a little over a year ago.

When he began he weighed 189 pounds. Two months later his weight had dropped very quickly to 175. It stayed there for the next three months—during a period when he stopped taking his daily two-mile fast walk.

Once he started walking again, he dropped on down to 170 pounds. He has remained there consistently ever since. Interestingly, this 170 pounds was the same weight he carried when he entered the Army some 40 years earlier.

In addition to the results with my friends, we also ran a three-week test with 22 people, 11 men and 11 women. In addition to the effect on their weight, we wanted to determine their attitudes toward the program.

Being new to *Zap the Fat*, they followed the program with varying degrees of consistency. Nevertheless, their results were quite consistent with our earlier observations.

Of the 22, 18 (8 men and 10 women) lost weight during the three weeks. Three of them (2 men and 1 woman) had no weight change. One man gained three pounds.

The average weight loss for those who lost weight was 4 1/2 pounds, or 1 1/2 pounds a week. The men averaged more (almost 2 pounds a week) than the women (over 1 pound a week), which was to be expected.

Their attitudes at the end of the program were generally consistent with their success. About 1 in 5 of them

(20%) said they definitely would not continue with the program. These included the one man who gained and two of the three who had no change in their weight.

Another 1 in 5 (20%) said that they definitely intended to adopt the program for their own on a life-time basis.

The remaining 3 in 5 (60%) said they would continue *Zap the Fat* in some ways, but were not ready to adopt it as a permanent life-style change.

This is the same as we had observed in the past among my friends. Of every five people who decided to try the program, one would reject it altogether, another would enthusiastically make the decision to change eating lifestyle this way for good, and three would realize it produced good results but were not ready to make the total commitment.

All those in the three-week test group were asked to tell what they particularly liked or disliked about *Zap the Fat*.

Leading the things they particularly liked about it, six people said they were never hungry and could eat all they wanted. Others were excited that they needed to count only *saturated* fat. Three stated they "did not need to think much about it" or "it was easy to follow."

Several told how it changed the way they feel. Some specific quotes:

- **"I like the way I feel now and my whole system seems to be functioning better."**

- **"I now feel excellent and like healthy, low-fat food better."**

- **"It is not a diet but a new way of life."**

- "It is easy to learn and identify the proper foods to eat."

- "Now I really have hopefulness regarding gradual weight loss."

Among the dislikes, five said giving up cheese was the hardest part. (Others said that substitution of non-fat cheese products such as cottage cheese, cream cheese and sour cream [see Chapter 4] made up for this very nicely.) Some had trouble giving up eggs, potato chips, fast food items, and various dairy products.

Others had a problem when eating out. And several mentioned trouble because everyone else in their household was not following the same program.

When asked whether they had learned anything from their three-week experiment, all but four answered yes. Again the negatives were the ones who had not benefited. It is unknown whether this resulted from failing to properly understand and follow the program, or for some other reason.

It was also interesting to note that half the 20% who were negative about the program and did not benefit from it, did not exercise. Since the simple exercise plan in Chapter 9 is an integral part of *Zap the Fat,* this would, of course, have had a negative effect on their results.

Once you make the decision to try *Zap the Fat,* you need to become familiar with the small number of foods that contain saturated fat. These will be described in this book.

These foods also are listed on the *Zap the Fat* Wallet Card. It fits easily into a wallet or purse. Soon you will be able to commit the list and saturated fat contents to memory. This is a short term project that can add years to your life and healthful pleasure to your years at the correct weight God meant you to carry.

One specific thing that must be given up completely is anything fried. Frying turns any fat into the equivalent of saturated fat. Assume that eating anything fried will use up more than 10 grams of saturated fat for that day. For me, the biggest hurdle was giving up fried foods.

I have cheated on this discipline two or three times during the past five years. And when I did, I chose some good old-fashioned Southern Fried Chicken. Each time I suffered with a stomach that rebelled at ingesting so much saturated fat after years of rest. Nor did it really taste as good as I had expected. It wasn't worth it.

There is one valuable principle that the *Zap the Fat* program uses to simplify lives. Since we have rounded the grams of saturated fat in items that we consume, all we need to do is to add to 10. No decimals or percentages. Just add the single digit figures for items eaten daily that contain saturated fat and make sure the total doesn't exceed 10.

No more calories to count. No exchanges to keep track of. No different types of fat to be concerned with.

As you have no doubt already judged, I am not a doctor. Nor a scientist. Nor a psychologist. This is not a medical or scientific or psychological book. It is merely my testimony of what I have discovered in living with the *Zap the Fat* eating program for more than five years. There is no guarantee that this will work for you. All I know is that it has worked for me, and for many of my friends.

At first glance, like all change, this may seem to be terribly difficult. I can only give you my testimony that for me it was not. There are so many good tasting substitutes without saturated fat today that it is just a matter of counting to 10 and developing new habit patterns.

3

CHANGING THE HABIT PATTERN

My experience with diets began when I was 30 years old. Until the time I married, my problem had been that I was too skinny.

In school I was always the last one chosen for any athletic team. My knobby knees were always kept hidden under a pair of long pants. I didn't like wearing a swimming suit, but for a different reason than most.

In fact, on the day I was married at the age of 20, I weighed 20 pounds less than what has proven to be my proper weight.

When I was 21, we moved to New York City where I took over management of an office with 100 people in it. I was just a year out of college with a set of very idealistic management ideas that didn't work very well when they were challenged by the domineering lady who was head of the union.

During the day I held all my feelings in since I certainly didn't want to create any waves. Occasionally I took it out on my poor wife at night. But since I had taken over the accounting and sales operation in addition to managing the office, there just wasn't time for that to happen very often either.

Two years later I developed an ulcer.

In those days treatment for an ulcer was simple. Eat

frequently. What I was told I must eat frequently contained a lot of saturated fat. Vast quantities of milk (today they have decided that is bad for ulcers!). Lots of cream cheese sandwiches. In fact, creamed anything.

The ulcer got better in a few months, but in the process I had developed an eating pattern that had already shot my weight up by more than 20 pounds. I had become quite comfortable with that new eating pattern. Except in the waist.

For the next seven years in New York I continued to put on weight. There were many wonderful places where we ate lunch. One I frequented about every other day specialized in desserts called Hortense's famous cream pies. I kid you not, those delicious creations stood a good six inches high.

So by my 30th birthday I was tipping the scales at 35 pounds over my proper weight—almost 25% more than it should be. The extra pounds sat loosely on my stomach and jowls.

That year two things happened that finally got my attention. First was a picture snapped of me at a gathering and published in a magazine. Could that fat face really be me? What a slob!

The second was simply the act of walking down stairs. I discovered that I was going down the stairs sideways—in order to keep my balance. My stomach rode so far out front that it was literally throwing me off balance whenever I tried to walk down stairs facing straight ahead.

So on my 30th birthday I decided to lose the extra pounds. In those days the fad diet was what they called the egg diet. Just eat eggs, in whatever form, and the protein will burn up the weight.

I ate up to a dozen eggs a day for a month. In all forms. And it worked. At least, it brought my weight down by 25 pounds. I was elated.

(Later, of course, I was to discover that this was the worst thing I could have done for my naturally high cholesterol level. I have often wondered how high my cholesterol level was at the end of those 30 days of continuous eggs.)

But of course, like all diets, the results were temporary. From time to time I would decide it was time to lose the five pounds I had gained. I'd start counting calories. But each time, of course, I looked forward daily to the end of the diet when I could get back to "normal" eating.

That is what differentiates the *Zap the Fat* eating program from any diet. This program is NOT a diet. It is a matter of changing a habit pattern.

I have a son-in-law who recently finished medical school. One day we were discussing the problems associated with changing habit patterns. It was something he had just been studying in depth, and he shed some light on the subject for me.

It seems that neurologists have discovered some very interesting things about our brains and how they relate to our habits. They point out that it takes at least 21 days for the brain to change any habit pattern.

The brain contains neurons and specialized supporting cells called neuroglia (nerve glue), or simply glia. The major function of glia is reception of information, integration of that information, generation of new signals, and transformation and conduction of messages. They can undergo cell division throughout adult life, and are responsible for the memory path that determines most of the things we do every day.

These glial cells are able to fire more rapidly when they are on a preferential path in our brains. Those preferential paths we have developed (usually many years ago) are the source of the habit patterns that govern our lives.

To change any one of these habit patterns is a major project. We must, in fact, establish a specific new pattern to replace the old one we have been comfortable with for so long.

And it isn't easy. We can't suddenly decide we will floss our teeth every day and just start doing it. We forget. Since we all view any change as some sort of loss, we rebel. So until we have firmly established that new habit pattern, we are in danger every day of just giving up what we have determined to change altogether.

The only way for that new path to develop in our brain is for us to follow a replacement pattern, consistently and consciously, for a period of at least 21 consecutive days.

It helped me to visualize a picture of a railroad switching yard. The yard has a number of different tracks, each of which goes to a different place. One of these tracks goes to Des Moines. Another goes to Topeka.

The Des Moines track has been used as the regular route for many years, but when the switch is moved so that the train will go over onto the Topeka track, the train heads for Topeka. It is the track that will be used from now on, as long as the switch is not changed back.

The Des Moines track is still there. It always will be. Grass may grow over it. May even cover it up. But it is still there.

It is only by 21 days of exclusive repetition of the new habit pattern that the new track can be laid. Once that is done, a brain will suppress the old track and use the new one. The old track is no longer the preferred route.

But directing something onto the new track for anything less than 21 days won't do it. Nor will trying to intersperse the new habit pattern with the old. We will be right back on the old habit pattern if we do not make a total commitment to the new one for the 21-day period.

Consequently, when we seriously adopt the *Zap the Fat* eating program and limit our intake of saturated fat to 10 grams per day for 21 consecutive days, we can accomplish the change in habit pattern. We can, and do, lay new track in our brains.

Part of that pattern is, of course, to consciously make the decision to adopt this as a lifetime method of eating. Not to think of it as a diet. To think "diet" guarantees disaster and an ultimate return to our same old roller coaster methods.

The danger of those methods has been demonstrated in several studies. One at the Cooper Institute for Aerobics Research in Dallas, Texas, was based on 12,025 Harvard University graduates with an average age of 67.

It found that more than twice as many (23.1%) of those who said they "always" dieted had heart disease compared with just 10.6% of those who answered they "never" dieted. Of those who dieted part of the time, the study found that the more they dieted, the higher their rates of heart disease.

Just before Christmas in 1985 I unexpectedly flew to London with my friend, Bobby Patterson. We had an appointment with an international organization regarding a Board on which I served.

We landed at Heathrow before dawn. Since our meeting in downtown London wasn't until ten o'clock, we decided to take the bus in.

It was one of those pay-on-the-bus deals. We boarded one that appeared out of the light mist with a couple of dozen other weary travelers who had been up all night.

We all took our seats while the cheerful driver started his routine of collecting the ticket fee.

He went to a woman in the first row and told her the amount due. She handed him a five pound note, thus requiring change. He made his way back to the front of the bus and made the change from one of those little mechanical holders designed to fit on his belt. Then he brought the change back to the lady along with her ticket.

He then turned to the man seated across the aisle from her and repeated the process. Then the next. Slowly he made his way toward the rear of the bus where we were seated.

After his fourth trip to the front for change and a ticket, I couldn't take it any longer. "Bobby," I exclaimed, "do you see that? Why doesn't he strap the change contraption on his belt and take the tickets in his hand? Then he could make change as he goes along and avoid all those trips back and forth. Do you realize how much time he is wasting?"

"Shut up," Bobby responded (I felt with more volume than necessary). "He's been doing it that way for at least 40 years and seems to be quite happy with it. Who asked you to help him change a habit of 40 years?"

We are faced first with a decision: do we want to change our habit pattern of many years standing? If so, we can establish a new habit pattern in our brain. It can and will create that new circuit. A new program makes it a habit to follow the way we need to eat.

Our lives can be changed forever. But only if we follow the action and the mindset of the *Zap the Fat* program for at least 21 consecutive days. Our brains can't create a new track any other way.

So what is the motivation to change our habit pattern?

Do we want to be free of diets forever? Do we want to be able to eat as much as we like and still arrive at and maintain our normal weight? Do we want to be healthier? Look better? Feel better?

Obviously, many of us do. That is why we diet. But by now we know that for most of us diets provide no lasting results. They never have. They never will.

If we are willing to make this lifetime decision, however, and spend 21 days developing the habit pattern, it can work for all of us—for a lifetime!

4

DAIRY & EGGS

As mentioned earlier, it's cheese that has always been my downfall. It didn't take me long to learn that ALL cheese has a lot of fat in it. But the discovery that two-thirds of that fat in cheese is saturated obviously spelled disaster for my old eating patterns.

What was I going to eat that could make up for a grilled cheese sandwich? Or what would an omelet be without some melted cheese pulling all those vegetables together? And who could imagine a bagel without a generous glob of cream cheese spread all over it?

I quickly realized that the relationship of all regular dairy products to *Zap the Fat* Eating was very simple: I could never eat any of them because they were all heavily made up of saturated fat.

That ruled out milk, cheese, ice cream, butter, any-thing creamed—just about everything worth eating.

But I knew it was a fact. There was no way to over-come the saturated fat problem unless I started with the decision to give up all regular dairy products. Forever!

Even though manufacturers often try to fool us with seemingly innocuous things like 1% milk or 2% milk, low-fat cheese and cottage cheese, "light" yogurt, etc., I can't rationalize the facts and fall for that temptation.

It's very simple. If there is ANY fat in a dairy product it is going to be primarily saturated fat and blows the whole program.

For example, an 8-ounce glass of so-called "2% milk" still contains 3 grams of saturated fat. And just a 1-ounce serving of what is labeled "low-fat" or "2%" cottage cheese contains the same 3 grams of saturated fat.

Butter is something else again. When I think of all the restaurant meals I complemented with four or five rolls slathered in creamy butter, it's enough to make me burp.

That's because just one little pat of butter (about one teaspoon) contains several grams of saturated fat. A tablespoon contains 7 grams. I was eating several day's allotment of the stuff in just one sitting! Small wonder my weight couldn't stay where it was supposed to be.

Or let's look at that health food mainstay: yogurt. A cup (8 ounces) of regular yogurt contains a whopping 5 grams of saturated fat. Even those labeled "low-fat" contain up to 3 grams of it.

And then there's ice cream. A normal serving (one cup) of regular ice cream (11% butterfat) contains 9 grams of saturated fat—almost a full day's allotment here, too. Even seemingly harmless sherbert contains a couple of grams.

Frozen yogurt is little better. It contains the same amount that you would find in regular yogurt—5 grams or so.

This discovery was a major depressant for me. We spend time every summer at a little town on Lake Michigan called Ludington. My family has been going there since my Dad was a year old in 1899. It's family.

It's also tradition. One of the main traditions is the old-fashioned ice cream store on Main Street. Since early childhood my vivid memories include almost daily visits to the House of Flavors to sample some tantalizing ice cream concoction such as the Pig's Dinner—if you ate it all you could wear a button that proudly declared you had succeeded in being a pig.

Consequently, I was crestfallen when I learned how much saturated fat there was in ice cream. And even in frozen yogurt. But my depression was short-lived when the next time in Ludington I found they had made a discovery that allowed me to again indulge myself in ice cream. It was non-fat ice cream. Five flavors!

This is illustrative of the big exception that alters, but does not eliminate, the dairy scene for us. A happy and important one. We may eat all we want of any dairy

DAIRY TABLE

To get an idea of why all dairy products (unless they are labeled NON-FAT) may not ever be eaten as part of our lifetime *Zap the Fat* program, note below the amount of saturated fat found in each of these representative items.

Item	Saturated Fat Grams
Ice Cream (11%) (1 cup)	9
Sherbert (1 cup)	2
Butter (tablespoon)	7
Parmesan Cheese (tablespoon)	1
American Cheese (1 oz slice)	6
(same applies to almost all other cheeses)	
Cottage Cheese (1 cup)	6
Cream Cheese (1 ounce)	6
Low-Fat Cheese (1 ounce slice)	3
Low-Fat (2%) Cottage Cheese (1 cup)	3
Milk (8 ounce glass/cup)	5
2% Milk (8 ounce glass/cup)	3
Light Coffee Cream (tablespoon)	2
Yogurt (1 cup)	5
Yogurt (Low-Fat or 2%) (cup)	3

product if it is labeled NON-FAT. Once we have com-mitted to memory these two words—NON-FAT—and adhere to their discipline, we have solved the dairy prob-lem for life. We will no longer have a problem with any dairy product.

If any dairy product is labeled non-fat, we may eat as much as we want. And today there is a proliferation of non-fat dairy products: cheese, cream cheese, cot-tage cheese, skim milk, ice cream, frozen yogurt, etc.

With all these new products as a starter, there are many substitutions we can use to make up for the satu-rated fat heavy dairy items that we can no longer eat.

BUTTER—What is a baked potato without butter? I have discovered it can be a number of things.

The most obvious is one of the non-saturated fat butter substitutes that come in shaker cans (e.g. Butter Buds). These are equally good on vegetables or sprinkled on just about anything that is heated.

Other baked potato coverings that are quite tasty are either salsa or shrimp cocktail sauce. Or even spicy chili beans (made without fat). At first such an order may turn up the eyebrows of a waitperson in a restau-rant when we are dining out. But I find places where I dine frequently soon start recommending my food or-ders to others.

If a baked potato seems inedible without sour cream we can still be in business. We can use the non-fat sour cream that, of course, contains no saturated fat. It's great alone or mixed with chopped chives or parsley.

Margarine without saturated fat is hard to come by, and therefore not a good option. There is at least one margarine (Promise Ultra Fat Free) that has absolutely no fat in it, however, and this is of course acceptable in any quantity. On those days we feel we absolutely must use up some of our day's allotment with margarine that does contain saturated fat, we should choose one that has no more than 2 grams, preferably less. That would include tub margarines or ones labeled "light" or "extra light." (See Chapter 6—Salad Dressings, Oils, and Margarine.)

Frankly, I found that, after my habit pattern was reversed, all breads, rolls, etc., on which I used to liberally spread margarine or butter were really quite tasty without it. Or without anything, for that matter.

In fact, one of the joys of this *Zap the Fat* method of eating is that we can eat all the bread we want without butter or margarine and we won't gain weight. I have often astonished my hosts or waitpersons by eating a half dozen rolls or pieces of bread at a sitting. "Aren't you afraid you'll gain weight?" they ask. I just smile.

CHEESE—There is no really good substitute for regular cheese, so it is necessary to begin by learning to live without it.

Pizza, for instance, is really excellent without any cheese on it at all. (That is the way it is normally prepared in much of southern France and northern Italy where it originated.)

Instead of cheese use extra pizza sauce. Then cover it liberally with the vegetables you like: olives (you do get a little saturated fat from them as noted in the Chapter 8 section on Fruits & Vegetables, so use them sparingly), artichoke hearts, broccoli, asparagus, mushrooms, green chiles, onions—and perhaps sprinkle a little garlic over the top along with some sun-dried tomatoes. No meat, of course, since all meat has some saturated fat. Those used on pizza are particularly high in it. Pizza is too good without meat to waste using up any of our saturated fat allotment for the day by adding it.

The pizza crust has at most negligible saturated fat, so we are free to consume as many pieces of one of these pizzas as we can handle. On the other hand, just one slice of a regular pizza with cheese can easily add up to a full day's allotment of saturated fat.

There is another answer to cheese. Non-fat (remember, "non," not just "low") cheeses are available in the grocery store. They come in different varieties including Swiss, American, mozzarella, and cheddar (which I find preferable to the others for both taste and melting factor). These don't have the full fat taste we remember from regular cheese, but they are getting better.

I make an acceptable grilled cheese sandwich with non-fat cheddar cheese. I cook it on low heat to provide time to melt. I like to put a lot of Dijon mustard on the bread, add some tomatoes or Ortega chile strips, and grill it in a skillet sprayed with Pam or a similar vegetable-based spray. The result: a quite good grilled cheese sandwich with no saturated fat. I usually eat at least two.

I've also found that a slice of non-fat American or cheddar cheese added to an omelet made with Egg Beaters, or similar egg substitute, makes for a great taste treat and satisfying meal. It melts very well on the direct heat on which the omelet is being cooked.

CREAM CHEESE—Kraft and Alpine Lace really had us in mind when they introduced their fat-free pasteurized process cream cheese product. Packed in a tub just like regular whipped cream cheese, it is great despite its somewhat long name (since it doesn't have fat the government won't let them call it just "cream cheese").

Unlike some other substitutes, this product is good used alone as well as in baked items or otherwise used as part of recipes. For example, we can make any of our favorite delicious cream cheese dips with it. I have a friend who bakes a marvelous cheese cake (see recipe in Desserts Addendum) using this product with skim milk.

These non-fat cream cheese type products are also excellent to spread on bagels or English muffins, or plain dry toast.

One other cream cheese substitute that I used before these new non-fat cream cheese products came out I make with non-fat yogurt. I take a 16-ounce container of plain (no flavor) yogurt. It must be the kind that contains no gelatin. Then I line a wire sieve with a piece of cheesecloth, put the yogurt on top of the cheesecloth, and place it over a 3-cup container in the refrigerator. Leave it to drain overnight.

The next morning all the liquid has drained into the container. Discard it. What remains on top of the cheesecloth is a mass the consistency of cream cheese. It has the same feel in the mouth and a very acceptable taste.

MILK—The answer here is skim milk, sometimes labeled non-fat milk. Remember, if it shows any percentage, even 1%, it contains saturated fat and should not be used. But skim milk is ALWAYS fine and works just as well in almost anything that calls for milk.

Evaporated skim milk can also be used when we want a creamier consistency such as in soups and sauces. If we get it very cold in the refrigerator we can even whip it. The result: whipped cream with no saturated fat.

For cooking, we get more thickness by using reconstituted dry non-fat skim milk. When used in cooking, one extra tablespoon of the dry milk is added to each cup of milk called for in the recipe.

We must be careful of so-called non-dairy cream

substitutes. They very often contain primarily coconut or palm oil (see Chapter 6 for their statistics)—as much as 12 grams of saturated fat in just one tablespoon. They are, in fact, almost nothing else.

ICE CREAM—With 9 grams or more of saturated fat per serving, regular ice cream is obviously out. But again, over the past few years, the manufacturers have created a broad substitute path we can follow.

Almost every grocery store today has one, and usually two or three, brands of non-fat (again not just low-fat) ice cream and frozen yogurt. They come in all flavors. Someone asked me once if they were really good. My response: when your alternative is none at all they are marvelous.

You can even make a saturated fat-free sundae using them. Most basic cook books have recipes for chocolate sauce made with just cocoa which contains no saturated fat (also see recipe in Desserts Addendum). Even Mrs. Richardson's famous ice cream toppings, such as hot fudge and butterscotch, now come in a non-fat version.

While these are things we can substitute for the fat-filled milk products we can't eat any more, remember they are not the only solution. We can always use any non-fat version of any dairy item and, regardless of quantity consumed, not add a single gram of our 10 gram daily allotment of saturated fat for that day.

Indeed, with all the options available to us, there is almost no reason to ever consume even one of our 10 grams a day of saturated fat by eating any dairy item other than those labeled non-fat.

EGGS—Egg yolks are a no-no in our program. While the white of the egg contains no saturated fat, the yolk contains 2 grams in each yolk. In addition the yolk is a primary culprit as a high cholesterol food (see Chapter 11 for details on cholesterol and sodium).

But this, too, is easy to get around. We actually have three choices available as substitutes:

- Use two egg whites every place it calls for a whole egg.
- Use any of the frozen packaged egg-substitutes found in the grocery store such as Egg Beaters, Second Nature, and Better'N Eggs. However, buying whole eggs and throwing away the yolks to get two egg whites used as an egg replacement is much cheaper than using the egg substitute. In fact, the cost usually works out to half as much for two whole egg whites as for the comparable amount of egg substitute.
- We can make our own egg substitute by mixing 2 egg whites with 1 teaspoon of non-fat powdered milk for each egg called for in a recipe. The yellow color can be replaced, if desired, with such things as saffron, tumeric, curry powder, yellow food coloring, or pureed carrots or squash (all depending, of course, on what we will be using the substitute).

Other than the obvious use of these substitutes for scrambled eggs or an omelet, there are countless other fine dishes that can be made with them: french toast, pancakes, waffles, even egg custards and other desserts that call for eggs.

We eat eggs in these forms several times a week. Not just for breakfast and desserts. We sometimes make pancakes, French toast, or waffles for dinner. They are every bit as satisfying as those made with whole eggs.

The message, then, on both dairy products and eggs is simple. We never eat any regular dairy product, whole eggs, or egg yolks. But we can eat all we want of any NON-FAT dairy products, egg whites, and egg substitutes.

We still have many exciting dairy items to eat that are non-fat and don't count at all toward our daily allotment of 10 grams of saturated fat. Isn't that our dream? To eat all we want and to know that we are not adding a single gram of saturated fat to our daily allotment, no matter how much of them we eat?

As for eggs, here too there are substitutes that mean we can eat almost anything we formerly ate that was made with whole eggs.

Actually, dairy and eggs are the easiest areas to comprehend. They're also the most fun to work with because of substitutes available. And, they're the least of the "will crossers," once we make up our mind to make the change away from all of them which contain saturated fat.

WALLET CARD SUMMARY

DAIRY and EGGS

Count 0 grams SF—NON-FAT Cheese, Cottage Cheese, Milk, Ice Cream, Yogurt, or any other milk product that is NON-FAT. Eat NO Butter.

Count 0 grams SF—Egg Whites or Egg Substitutes.
Count 2 grams SF—a whole egg or egg yolk.

5

ALL ABOUT MEAT

During my five-week stay at Massachusetts General Hospital, I was required to attend twice-weekly discharge classes. Often I got into quite heated discussions with that diminutive Korean dietician who conducted them all.

At the time it seemed to me that I lost some and won some. In retrospect, I maybe won a point once or twice. Usually I was no match for her.

One particular subject that I pursued with her many times was bacon. I love bacon. Bacon is to die for. What lunch is as satisfying as a marvelous bacon, lettuce and tomato sandwich? Even Egg Beaters might be bearable—but live without even one slice of bacon?

Toward the end of my stay there I was feeling better and more feisty. One day she and I really had it out. All over a piece of bacon. Just one.

"Couldn't I have just one on occasion?"

I explained patiently how I cook my bacon.

"You see, I like my bacon crisp. I mean really crisp. I cook it until ALL the fat is cooked away.

"Then I drain it on paper towels—and not just one paper towel, either. I place one on the bottom and another on top of the cooked bacon. Then I press it lovingly, using those paper towels to soak up every bit of

49

fat that may have been left clinging to that crisp morsel."

After listening to me ramble on about the mouth-watering virtue of MY bacon with all the fat blotted away, my dietician friend rose up to her full 4-foot 9-inch height.

She put her hands on her hips and spat at me just like one of those sputtering pieces of bacon: "Mr. French! Mr. French! You must understand. Bacon is all fat. All fat! There is nothing else in it but fat. If there is ANYTHING left over after you finish with it, that is fat. YOU MAY NOT HAVE BACON."

Needless to say, I really learned my lesson that day. I learned it so well that I would never let myself think about bacon for several years.

Even when I started using the *Zap the Fat* eating method and began concentrating solely on the saturated fat in what I ate. I still didn't let myself consider whether bacon might now be acceptable. I had trained myself as well as Pavlov's famous dog.

That continued until not long ago. But one day when I was studying the tables I spotted an amazing truth.

The saturated fat in a cooked piece of bacon is just 1 gram! Since I usually consume two or three of my 10 grams per day at the noon meal, this meant that I could now lunch on two bacon, lettuce, and tomato sandwiches made with one piece of bacon in each and saturated fat-free mayonnaise and still have eaten just two of my 10 gram allotment for the day. Yes, I could have bacon after all!

(It is interesting to note that "turkey bacon" has almost the same amount of saturated fat after cooking as regular bacon. I personally don't find the turkey variety nearly as tasty as the pork product.)

Meat will cost most of us about half, or more, of our

daily 10 gram saturated fat allotment. Consequently, unless we become vegetarians, it is the area to which we need to devote the most attention.

From all I had read, I had begun to get the feeling that red meat was best eliminated from my diet. But as I looked at it more carefully, it was exciting to discover that I did not need to give up red meat altogether. Indeed, as our Beef and Veal Table shows, I could eat 3 ounces a day of red meat and still have 7 grams of saturated fat left over to apply to other things.

BEEF and VEAL TABLE

(with all visible fat removed)

(All figures are for 3-ounce portions [size of a deck of cards] unless otherwise noted.)

Item	Saturated Fat Grams
Sirloin Steak	2
Brisket	3
Flank Steak	3
London Broil	3
New York Steak	3
Porterhouse Steak	3
Round Steak	3
T Bone Steak	3
Tenderloin	3
Ribs, Beef or Pork (1 rib)	4
Veal Cutlet	4
Chuck	5
Hamburger	7

For the purposes of our tables and our *Zap the Fat* Wallet Card, the portion size we use for meat of all varieties is usually 3 ounces. This is because that is a size that is easy to identify, since a 3-ounce portion of meat can be compared to the size of a deck of cards. This makes it easy to equate our portion size with the saturated fat in what we are eating.

Therefore, I try to make sure I limit my consumption to a piece of meat no larger than a deck of cards. Then I can tell from the numbers shown in the table the amount of saturated fat I am eating. If I eat a piece twice that size I know I need to double the number of grams.

For example, the Beef and Veal Table shows a 3-ounce portion of most cuts of beef means that I have consumed 3 grams of saturated fat. Eat a piece the size of two decks of cards and I have doubled the saturated fat to 6 grams, a very high percentage of my day's allotment to use on just one item.

By comparison, if I eat the same deck of cards-sized piece of white meat of chicken without skin, or of most fish, I have only consumed 1 gram of saturated fat. Double that portion and I still have only had 2 grams. In fact, I could eat a whopping 3 card deck-sized piece of chicken white meat without any skin and still equal what I would get from a one deck-sized piece of beef. This is why fish and chicken are normally preferred over red meat.

One beef problem I learned about quickly was hamburger. Indeed, a normal quarter pounder hamburger bought at the grocery store or purchased at a fast food restaurant is going to contain almost 10 grams of saturated fat. That's just a 4-ounce piece of cooked meat.

Like bacon, my first reaction was to give up hamburger all together. But that wasn't all that was affected. Giving up hamburger also meant changing the way I cooked things like chili. And spaghetti. I couldn't put any ground beef in them either. What a bummer.

Then the light dawned. Under the *Zap the Fat* program this is not necessarily the case. It just takes careful buying and conservative use.

It's quite easy to accomplish. First, I purchase sirloin steak (just 2 grams of saturated fat in a 3-ounce portion) or round steak (just 3 grams of saturated fat in the same sized portion). Then I have the butcher trim off all the visible fat. Then I ask him to grind it for me just as he would hamburger.

I end up with meat that contains just 3 grams of saturated fat in a card deck size portion. It can then be shaped as a hamburger.

(In selecting beef at your grocers, always look for that which is labeled "Choice." All figures in our Beef and Veal Table assume we have purchased "Choice" and not "Prime" beef. "Prime" contains much more "marbling," which is actually just fat. There is also a grade called "Select" which has even less fat than "Choice," but it is not worth the sacrifice of flavor since it produces only a minor saving in saturated fat.)

There are other things you can do with ground sirloin or round steak that can be even more exciting.

We had started making and eating (without much joy) vegetarian chili and spaghetti sauce. Frankly, they just didn't cut it. In fact, I found them mighty dull and tasteless, although my wife, who is more a vegetable lover than I am, thought they were OK.

Once we realized the numbers on ground sirloin we tried an experiment. To that vegetarian chili or spaghetti sauce we added a single 3-ounce hamburger patty made with the ground sirloin steak.

The results were amazing. Just one little 3-ounce patty brought the sauce back to life. It regained the feel and taste of our old chili and spaghetti sauces.

When I reviewed the figures I really thought I'd died and gone to heaven. Not only did it taste great, but the

LAMB, PORK, POULTRY, LUNCH MEATS, and GAME TABLE

(with all visible fat removed)

(All figures are for 3-ounce portions [size of a deck of cards] unless otherwise noted.)

Item	Saturated Fat Grams
Bacon (1 slice, cooked)	1
Chicken (white) w/o skin	1
Turkey (white) w/o skin	1
Buffalo	1
Elk	1
Rabbit	1
Venison	1
Pork Tenderloin	2
Chicken (dark) w/o skin	2
Turkey (dark) w/o skin	2
Boar	2
Lamb Loin	3
Chicken (white) with skin	3
Turkey (white) with skin	3
Bologna (1 ounce slice)	3
Dove	3
Duck (wild-without skin)	3
Pheasant	3
Quail	3
Lamb Chop	4
Chicken (dark) with skin	4
Turkey (dark) with skin	4
Duck (domestic without skin)	4
Goose	4
Ham	5
Hot Dog (1 regular size)	5
Pork Chop	7
Chicken - Fried	7

recipe produced four large servings. That meant that each serving contained less than 1 gram of saturated fat!

Serve it with some french bread and a salad smothered with non-fat dressing. The result: a complete and very satisfying meal that has used up only 1 gram of saturated fat. Nine left that I can still eat that day.

I have also learned that there are many quality meat products in the average supermarket that replace those eliminated because of their saturated fat content.

For example, take hot dogs. As our table shows, a single regular sized hot dog contains at least 5 grams of saturated fat. This is the case whether it has been made with beef, pork, chicken, or turkey. Hot dogs just naturally contain way too much saturated fat for our program.

But hot dogs did not need to be eliminated from my diet altogether. A careful search in the hot dog case revealed that there are now at least two brands (Hormel's Light & Lean and Healthy Choice) that contain only 1/2 gram or less of saturated fat in each hot dog. And they still taste good. Very good, in fact.

I could now eat a couple of these hot dogs on buns for lunch. Complete with mustard, ketchup, pickles, onions—the works. And still have consumed only one countable gram of saturated fat, since the buns contain no saturated fat grams (See Chapter 7).

But if I had picked the regular variety from the case, those same two hot dogs would have put me over the top for the day.

Dieting is a hard habit to break. I have to keep reminding myself that all I am to count is saturated fat. I do not have to be concerned with, or even know, how many calories there are in the hot dog, the ketchup, the mustard, the pickles, or even the bun.

Whatever contains no saturated fat contains nothing that has any bearing on the program.

FISH TABLE

(All figures are for 3-ounce portions [size of deck of cards] unless otherwise noted.)

All of the following have NO countable saturated fat and need not be counted at all:

Clams	Perch
Cod	Rockfish
Crab	Sand Dabs
Flounder	Scallops
Grouper	Scrod
Haddock	Sea Bass
Halibut	Shrimp
Lobster	Snapper
Mahi Mahi	Sole
Mussels	Tuna (packed in water)
Northern Pike	

The following are the fish which do need to be counted:

Item	Saturated Fat Grams
Bluefish	1
Catfish	1
Mackerel	1
Orange Roughie	1
Oysters	1
Salmon	1
Trout	1
Tuna (packed in oil)	1
Whitefish	1
Anchovies	2
Herring	2
Sardines	2
Shark	2
Swordfish	2
Pompano	4

As far as my weight control program is concerned, I have eaten nothing that counts against my daily saturated fat allotment. NO SATURATED FAT = NO COUNT!

Another problem is packaged lunch meats. They are often heralded with advertising slogans like "97% fat free." This doesn't mean much to us. A piece of bologna is still 3 grams of saturated fat in just a single 1-ounce slice—much less than is normally used on a sandwich.

We must always check the labels on packaged meats. They show how much saturated fat is in a portion. Then we need to check the portion to be sure it is the amount we will be eating.

We must decide if we are going to be happy with the specified portion in a sandwich or for a meal. If not, we must increase our count based on the quantity we will be consuming.

No matter what percentage of "fat free" is shown, almost all packaged lunch meats contain at least 1 gram of saturated fat per slice. I finally decided they couldn't work for me and gave up eating any of these pre-packaged lunch meats at all.

And next I found the most pleasantly surprising area of all: fish. As noted in the Fish Table, there is NO countable saturated fat in a three-ounce portion of many kinds of fish, including almost all shell fish.

That means there is nothing to count against your day's allotment when you eat such popular fish as snapper, mahi mahi, halibut, flounder, cod, and tuna (packed in water—if it is packed in oil it does count as 1 gram per card deck-sized serving). You don't have to count any saturated fat from these fish no matter how much of them you eat.

Shell fish which also count as NO saturated fat at all

include just about everything—you never have to count saturated fat against your daily allotment when you eat crab, clams, lobster, mussels, shrimp, or scallops. Nothing counts from any shell fish except oysters.

Choosing the type of meat I am going to eat is just half the battle, however. The other half is how I cook it. That is what determines whether I am adding more saturated fat than was in the meat itself.

For example, if I fry any meat—even a piece of white meat of chicken—its normal 3 grams of saturated fat in a 3-ounce portion with skin jumps to as much as 7 grams of saturated fat. In that same piece of chicken. This is why frying ANYTHING is out for life. It just does not fit into our diet.

(Incidentally, there has been a lot of misinformation about preparing chicken and turkey. Eating the skin doubles the saturated fat, that is true. However, it is not necessary to remove the skin before baking or broiling. As long as the skin is removed before eating, the extra saturated fat is gone.)

Instead of frying there are a wide variety of cooking options available to us. Bake it. Boil it. Broil it. Braise it. Grill it. Poach it. Roast it. Steam it. Stew it.

But do NOT use butter for any of these methods of cooking. A little canola oil is OK (no more than a tablespoon per serving). But even that will add 1 gram of saturated fat to the total for the meal.

Another approach is to saute. Even though "saute" is a French word meaning to "fry in very little oil." Just use a little wine or broth. Or prepare the skillet with one of the several types of vegetable cooking sprays that are available (probably the best known is Pam). You can also still stir fry, using those same vegetable sprays.

Flavor is also improved by marinading in wine with herbs. Or try using lemon, fruit juices, and spices. Or saute in chicken or beef broth. Even fat-free salad dressings. There are so many different way to enhance the flavor of meat, poultry, and fish dishes without adding more fat.

We need to use the tables to determine the amount of saturated fat in the meat, poultry, fish, and game we are eating. I find it best never to eat anything that will add up to more than 3 grams of saturated fat, or less than a third of a day's allotment.

You will find we have not included any organ meats in the tables. This is because they have too much cholesterol to be included in anyone's diet. All of the meats, poultry, and fish that are included can be assumed to contain approximately 75 milligrams of cholesterol in a 3-ounce portion. The only exception to this is shrimp, which contain about 45 milligrams per ounce, or 135 in a 3-ounce portion.

As we continue, we will discover there are many exciting things to learn about meats, poultry, and fish. Some we can eat without having to count anything against our daily allotment of saturated fat at all. Others we can eat in 3-ounce portions and add just one or two grams of saturated fat to our daily consumption.

But we must always be alert to a few things:

- Portion size should be equal to that of a deck of cards.
- Nothing should ever be fried.
- Everything should always be cooked without butter.
- If we add oil when cooking, its saturated fat must also be counted (see Chapter 6)—e.g. two grams for each tablespoon of olive oil.

WALLET CARD SUMMARY

MEAT, POULTRY and FISH

SATURATED FAT (SF) CONTENT FOR ALL = 3-ounce portion (size of a deck of cards), with all fat or skin removed, unless otherwise noted.

MEATS
Count 1 gram SF—Bacon (1 slice), Buffalo, Elk, Rabbit, Venison.

Count 2 grams SF—Pork Tenderloin, Sirloin Steak, Boar.

Count 3 grams SF—Brisket, Flank Steak, London Broil, New York Steak, Porterhouse Steak, Round Steak, T Bone Steak, Tenderloin, Lamb Loin.

POULTRY
Count 1 gram SF—White Chicken, White Turkey

Count 2 grams SF—Dark Chicken, Dark Turkey

FISH
Count 0 grams SF—Clams, Cod, Crab, Flounder, Grouper, Haddock, Halibut, Lobster, Mahi Mahi, Mussels, Northern Pike, Perch, Rockfish, Sand Dabs, Scallops, Scrod, Sea Bass, Shrimp, Snapper, Sole, Tuna (fresh or packed in water).

Count 1 gram SF—Bluefish, Catfish, Mackerel, Orange Roughie, Oysters, Salmon, Trout, Tuna (packed in oil), Whitefish.

Count 2 grams SF—Anchovies, Herring, Sardines, Shark, Swordfish.

6

SALAD DRESSINGS, OILS, & MARGARINE

"I want a toikey sannich on round sannich bread with lettuce and lots and lots of maynaise."

I was maybe four years old. But my will had already been quite well set. I knew what I liked. Whenever I was asked what I wanted to eat it was always that same "toikey sannich made on round sannich bread and with lots and lots of maynaise."

In one way my dietary restrictions today have been made easier by that habit pattern developed so many years ago. At least I hadn't set my heart on a ham and Swiss cheese sandwich. Or corned beef. Or roast beef.

But the problem created by that old habit pattern was, of course, what else I put on my turkey sandwich. The turkey itself, even when I heaped on a full three ounces of white meat, used up just one gram of my saturated fat allotment for the day.

SALAD DRESSINGS

But that mayonnaise! When I apply mayonnaise to a sandwich it is like putting grease on a rusted bolt. I slather both pieces of bread with a couple of tablespoons of that marvelous, rich dressing. Regardless of what kind of sandwich I may be creating.

Unfortunately, each of those tablespoons contributes 2 grams of saturated fat to my daily total. Just one of my sandwiches added another 8 grams of saturated fat because of my freedom with those four tablespoons of mayonnaise.

There are many other things that seem to taste right only when mayonnaise is a part of their make-up. Several tablespoons of mayonnaise.

Take a grilled cheese and tomato sandwich, for instance. Or a tomato aspic salad. How about tuna salad, either eaten in a sandwich or served on a crisp bed of lettuce as a salad? And what would Thanksgiving be without a turkey sandwich made from the leftovers before you go to bed?

Our Salad Dressing Table shows us that mayonnaise provides two grams of saturated fat for each tablespoon we use. Fortunately, however, thanks to the wonders of modern food manufacturing there is hope for us junkies who must count our saturated fat.

The major manufacturers took their first step by cutting the saturated fat in what they called "light" mayonnaise. The saturated fat was cut to just 1 gram.

Then Kraft came along with a totally non-fat mayonnaise—not only did it have no saturated fat, but it had no fat at all. Unfortunately, this non-fat offering just doesn't give me any of the feel of real mayonnaise since it contains no fat at all. By itself, it just is not a viable substitute in my eyes or mouth. My wife, however, finds it quite acceptable on sandwiches when mixed half and half with ketchup for a non-fat type Thousand Island dressing.

One little-known manufacturer has, in my opinion, found the right solution for those of us involved in the *Zap the Fat* program. Their product is called Nalley's Light Mayonnaise. (If you don't find it in your supermarket ask them to order it for you: Nalley's Fine Foods,

Division of Curtice Burns Foods, Tacoma, Washington 98411.) It contains 5 grams of total fat, but NONE of that is saturated. Weight Watchers also has a good tasting Light Mayonnaise with no saturated fat and only 2 grams of fat. These compare with the other "light" mayonnaises which have just five grams of total fat, but one of those grams is saturated. Regular mayonnaise, of course, has 11 grams of total fat and two of those are saturated.

SALAD DRESSING TABLE

(All figures shown are for one tablespoon of dressing.)

Item	Saturated Fat Grams
Mayonnaise, non-fat or Nalley's or Weight Watchers' Light	0
Mayonnaise, light	1
Caesar	1
Italian	1
Thousand Island	1
Ranch	1
Mayonnaise, regular	2
Blue Cheese	2
French	2

Besides saturated fat-free mayonnaise, there are other exciting things that can be used on sandwiches. A friend of mine has one that he calls George's Potion. It is quite easy to make.

He starts with yogurt cheese which he makes by draining non-fat yogurt over cheese cloth as explained in Chapter 4. To three parts of this yogurt cheese he adds one part of mustard. Or, when he wants a stronger concoction, he uses one part prepared mustard to just two parts of the yogurt cheese.

He uses almost any kind of mustard. Normally it's Dijon and it is marvelous. Sometimes he adds variety by using a different type—honey mustard, regular brown, special hot, etc. Whatever type of mustard, George's Potion really dresses up a sandwich.

Of course, a more obvious and simpler substitute is to use mustard alone. Or ketchup.

OILS

It is not only mayonnaise that we must be careful with, however. All oils—and therefore all salad dressings that are made with oil—contain one or two grams of saturated fat in each tablespoon (see Oils Table).

OILS TABLE

(All figures shown are for one tablespoon of the oil listed.)

Item	Saturated Fat Grams
Almond	1
Canola	1
Safflower	1
Sunflower	1
Walnut	1
Corn	2
Olive	2
Peanut	2
Sesame	2
Soybean	2
Cottonseed	4
Palm	7
Palm Kernel	11
Coconut	12

One way to overcome the problem is by using one of the many varieties of fat-free salad dressings now found in the supermarket. Richard Mayer, the chairman of Kraft Foods, was quoted as saying that fully 30% of the Kraft salad dressings that were sold in 1993 were fat free.

Personally, I have not yet found a fat-free salad dressing that I really enjoy. Instead, I find using a couple of tablespoons of salad dressing made with one of our single gram saturated fat oils (almond, canola, safflower, sunflower, or walnut) is one of those times when it's worth it to me to use up two grams of my daily saturated fat allotment.

I also like to experiment with different ways to make salad dressings from scratch.

For a creamy dressing, I start with non-fat yogurt. Or non-fat cottage cheese. After whipping them in the blender, there are a multitude of tastes that can be created by adding different seasonings, e.g. dill weed, horseradish, curry, or fruit juice.

A closer look at the Oils Table reveals some surprises about the various types. Particularly noteworthy are palm oil, palm kernel oil, and coconut oil. As little as just one tablespoon of any of these three oils can use up a whole day's allotment of saturated fat and then some.

Since palm, palm kernel, and coconut oils are often used in packaged products, it is a good idea always to read labels and make a point never to buy anything made with any of them.

Particularly watch out for cookies and crackers made overseas. Manufacturers there still use these highly saturated fat oils freely, because they prolong the shelf life of a product containing them. Most American manufacturers have eliminated them from their products.

Among the worst offenders made in this country are non-dairy creamers. Many are still made with either coconut or palm oil.

There is another reason we need to be on guard about anything containing palm, palm kernel, or coconut oils. Packaging can be misleading because of the portion size designated.

One well-known brand of whipped topping, for example, is made with coconut and palm oils. It brags on the label that it "contains no saturated fat in a serving." But closer scrutiny reveals that the serving size they are referring to is just two tablespoons.

One time my wife used several times that much of this product for a cake topping. She proudly showed me the box that stated a serving contained no saturated fat. But the amount of it used for my piece of cake was a different story. Since the primary ingredients were two of these saturated-fat heavy oils, there were several grams of saturated fat on my single piece of cake.

It is therefore better to stay away from anything that contains any palm, palm kernel, or coconut oils.

MARGARINE

Back in Chapter 4 we made a detailed exploration of butter. The conclusion was the need to eliminate butter from our diets altogether if we are following the *Zap the Fat* program. Using any butter at all almost guarantees that we will exceed our 10 grams of saturated fat for a day.

But what about margarine? While 70% of the fat in butter is saturated, only about 10% of the fat in regular stick margarine is.

So margarine is always considerably better that butter. But even though it is always much lower in saturated fat than butter, margarine can be tricky also.

There is a simple rule of thumb to help us. The harder the margarine is in consistency, the higher it is going to be in saturated fat.

MARGARINE TABLE

(All figures shown are for one tablespoon of margarine.)

Item	Saturated Fat Grams
Fat Free	0
Liquid	1
Tub	1
Stick (solid)	2

This is because manufacturers hydrogenate the unsaturated fat used in making margarine so that it will become more solid. This hydrogenation actually turns formerly unsaturated fat into saturated fat. The same sort of thing that happens when you fry something.

This is true even for margarines that say the oil used is just "partially hydrogenated." Any oil which is hydrogenated at all is bad for those of us trying to follow the *Zap the Fat* program.

As we see in the Margarine Table, there are 2 grams of saturated fat in a tablespoon of regular, stick margarine. When we choose to use softer margarines, such as those which come in tubs, that saturated fat is cut in half.

Thanks again to the wonders of modern manufacturing, there is now at least one margarine which is the best for our program. It not only tastes pretty good, but it contains absolutely no saturated fat at all.

It is named Ultra Fat Free from Promise (not to be confused with other Promise margarines which contain some saturated fat). Other manufacturers are sure to follow with their versions of similar saturated fat-free margarines.

Package labels are now required by the Food and Drug Administration (FDA) to designate the saturated fat content of margarine products. Look for margarines that list liquid oil as the first ingredient. Or, if the first ingredient is water, then liquid oil should be the second ingredient.

These so-called diet margarines are great for spreading. However, because of their water content, they are quite difficult, if not impossible, to use for cooking. Use canola oil as a substitute.

ANOTHER SPREAD

In addition to the use of low-fat margarine or any of the other fat-free spreads we have covered (no pun intended), I couldn't close without mentioning my very favorite.

Slice the top off a couple of garlic bulbs, about a half-inch from the top. Wrap them in aluminum foil and bake them for 35 minutes at 375 degrees.

Now, take a few tablespoons of that non-fat yogurt cheese (see Chapter 5). Squeeze the soft garlic flesh out of the roasted skin and mash it in with the yogurt cheese. Add other seasonings to taste such as pepper, rosemary, juniper berries–but nothing to overwhelm the garlic flavor.

This creates another marvelous spread to use on bread or rolls. Some Italian restaurants today are providing this spread to be used in place of butter or olive oil.

You can also spread just the baked garlic on bread.

All this can be a lot of fun. We don't have to give up good eating just because we need to change our eating habit pattern. We can cut out the majority of the saturated fat in our diets and still eat very well.

Indeed, what we use to replace that harmful saturated fat can turn out to be even better than what we started with. It's all a matter of attitude.

WALLET CARD SUMMARY

SALAD DRESSINGS, OILS, MARGARINE

SATURATED FAT (SF) PER TABLESPOON

SALAD DRESSINGS
Count 0 grams SF—Non-Fat or Nalley's or Weight Watchers "Light" Mayonnaise
Count 1 gram SF—Caesar, Italian, Thousand Island, Ranch, other "Light" Mayonnaise
Count 2 grams SF—Blue Cheese, French, Roquefort, Regular Mayonnaise

OILS
Count 1 gram SF—Almond, Canola, Safflower, Sunflower, Walnut.
Count 2 grams SF—Corn, Olive, Peanut, Sesame, Soybean

MARGARINE
Count 0 grams SF—labeled "Fat Free" or "Non-fat"
Count 1 gram SF—Liquid, Tub
Count 2 grams SF—Stick or Solid

7

BREADS, DESSERTS, & CANDY

We eat out frequently. Do most of our entertaining at restaurants. I like to be waited on. To enjoy food served on fine china. It's interesting to look over the variety of things on the menu and to share with our friends without the distractions of my own kitchen.

We always try to make it a festive occasion. But that can be a problem for me. I have a tendency to overeat. That was sometimes a disaster until I discovered the magic of bread.

BREADS

Regular restaurant rolls, french bread, bread sticks—in fact, just about any type of bread the normal restaurant puts out on the table—contain no measurable saturated fat. Consequently, I can eat all of them I want. And I do!

My problem is created by the average waiter. He brings us a basket of rolls for the whole table and assumes his bread duties for the evening are concluded as far as our table is concerned.

But not at my table! Little does he know that I am going to eat more than the bread in that basket. All by myself. We'll be needing at least another basket for the rest of the people dining with me. Unless any of them are also on the *Zap the Fat* program, in which case we'll need several more baskets!

When things get really sticky, however, is at one of those restaurants where they pass you one roll at a time. The bus boy wanders around from time to time plopping one on your butter plate.

The first time he appears, I ask him to please skip the butter or margarine he starts to place on my butter plate.

Then he interprets the fact I don't want any butter or margarine as meaning I won't be eating the roll he left either. So he disappears. He sees no need to come back and check to see if I want any more. But of course, not taking butter or margarine has nothing to do with what I am going to do to those rolls.

To make up for the disappearing act on the part of the roll boy, my poor wife has an ongoing instruction from me. It is to apply whenever and wherever we eat out. She is never, never, never to let that waitperson get past her without getting another roll on her butter plate.

"Even if you have to ask him for it, get it. Even though you do not want any more yourself, get one. Rest assured, I will eat it. This way, each time he passes the table we can increase the ante by two rolls."

So why all the fuss about bread and rolls? Because they have been so maligned over the years as something we must watch out for in order to control our weight. Instead, in the *Zap the Fat* program we can eat all of them we want without affecting our saturated fat count at all.

In addition to any kind of bread—white, whole wheat, french, sourdough, etc.—this includes hard rolls, french rolls, and bread sticks. As well as all the bagels and English muffins we can eat. They add a total zero to our intake of saturated fat for the day.

NO-COUNT BREAD PRODUCTS TABLE

(All the following have no countable saturated fat content and are counted as 0 Saturated Fat.)

Bagels (except Egg Bagels which are NOT OK)
Bread - White
Bread - Whole Wheat
Bread - French
Bread - Sourdough
Bread Sticks (Plain)
Buns (Hamburger or Hot Dog)
English Muffins
Rolls - Hard or Soft
Rolls - French

The thing we still cannot do, of course, is to put anything with fat on these bread items. No butter. No margarine. No olive oil and garlic mixture. All of these add varying amounts of saturated fat, particularly if you eat as many rolls or pieces of bread as I do.

But the breads themselves are saturated fat-free as far as our program is concerned. We can eat as much of any of them as we want!

Of course, we can opt to use some of our 10-gram saturated fat allotment for the day by putting spread on our bread. Personally, once the habit pattern was developed I discovered that all bread and rolls taste very good by themselves. I don't feel any need to dress them up with saturated fat-loaded spreads.

When I am eating at home and want to put something on them, however, all is still not lost. Non-fat cream cheese goes great with jelly on bagels or English muffins. The non-fat Promise Ultra margarine can also be used. Or we can try a spread like apple butter. None of these will add any saturated fat to our count at all.

Just remember, butter is out (7 grams of saturated fat to the tablespoon).

While all these bread products are saturated fat-free for us, quite the opposite is the case with almost everything else that is baked. In fact, as we will note from the Baked Goods Fat Table, with very few exceptions we must eliminate other regular baked products altogether.

DESSERTS

I grew up during the depression. Consequently, we ate what we considered to be quite simple and wholesome meals. I remember fondly the "simple" Sunday evening suppers at Aunt Lois' home. They were the same every Sunday.

The meal was centered around a couple of waffles for each of us. Real, old fashioned, home made waffles. Each batch of batter was made with several eggs, 6 or 7 tablespoons of butter, and a cup and a half of whole milk.

Then we would pour melted butter over each waffle from the big pitcher that sat in the middle of the table. Always enough to fill each little indentation to the brim. Then we'd slop on the maple syrup.

And, of course, there were always several pieces of bacon to give an added crispness to our simple supper.

I realize now that my "simple" supper contained somewhere between 30 and 40 grams of saturated fat. An entire three to four days allotment!

Another example is a danish. It can exceed a full day's allotment. Or how about a piece of cheesecake, which tops the chart at 22 grams of saturated fat—more than the amount we can eat in two days? (A saturated fat-free recipe for Chocolate Cheesecake is found in the Addendum.)

Of course, when we are baking at home it's a different story. We have already discovered there are a number of ways we can greatly decrease, and in some cases eliminate all together, the saturated fat in things such as waffles, cakes, pies, etc. just by substituting NON-FAT ingredients for those normally used.

BAKED GOODS TABLE

(Saturated fat for normal-sized serving unless otherwise noted.)

Item	Saturated Fat Grams
Crackers - Graham (2)	1
Crackers - Saltines (6)	1
Pancakes (2) 4" diameter	1
Popover	1
Biscuit	2
Brownie	2
Chocolate Chip Cookie	2
Muffin - Bran	2
Muffin - Corn	2
Cornbread	3
Doughnut - Cake	3
Muffin - Carrot	3
Sweet Roll	4
Muffin - Blueberry	4
Pie - Fruit	4
Doughnut - Glazed	5
Pie - Pumpkin	7
Cake - Pound	7
Croissant	7
Pie - Cream	8
Cake - Chocolate	9
Waffle (9" diameter)	4 to 9
Danish	11
Cheesecake	22

In fact, about the only things that just won't taste as good when we alter their recipes to make them saturated fat-free are croissants, doughnuts (because they are fried and that is what gives them their taste) and some cookies.

On the bright side, let's take fruit pies as an example. The main culprit in any pie is the fat in its crust. To make it even worse, most commercially baked pies contain lard in that crust. But we can make crust with canola oil and cut the saturated fat back to an acceptable level.

We can even work wonders with cream pies. Obviously it is the milk in them that provides the saturated fat. Instead of whole milk we can use canned evaporated skim milk and get the same rich feel and taste. Or use the non-fat packaged puddings that come in several delicious flavors.

This even works for cheesecake. A normal piece carries a whopping 22 grams of saturated fat. But we make one that uses crushed graham crackers for the crust. The filling is then made with non-fat cream cheese and egg whites. (See Desserts in Addendum.) Other ingredients remain the same. But the saturated fat drops from those 22 grams in a serving to no countable amount. Zero instead of 22. Yet it still tastes very good.

The same applies to cakes and cookies, such as brownies. One excellent fat substitute we use in baking is applesauce. Or substitute a puree of some other type of fruit such as prunes or banana, combined with a little water. The puree taste is not noticeable. Use these purees to replace the oil, butter, or margarine called for in the recipe. Without losing any flavor or substance.

When it comes to chocolate there is an alternative for us. The secret is to avoid milk chocolate or unsweetened baking chocolate. As well as anything containing cocoa butter. They are what provide the saturated fat.

Instead make chocolate dishes using regular cocoa powder, either sweetened or unsweetened, which contains no saturated fat. Use non-fat milk or canned evaporated skim milk in place of whole milk; a fruit puree instead of butter, margarine, and oils; and two egg whites to replace each whole egg called for in a recipe.

This has become a community experience. Along with several friends who live close by, we like to experiment with new recipes. When one is a success we share the results with one another. This is particularly true with desserts. You will find several of those which have been born this way in the dessert recipes at the end of the book.

When we don't have time to do the baking ourselves, there are more and more good-tasting, yet saturated fat-free, options available today in the supermarket.

The lead in developing really excellent tasting yet fat-free cakes, cookies, and coffee cakes was taken back in 1990 by Entenmann's. Today, almost every grocery store has a section devoted to their non-fat baked goods. By mid-1993, more than 25% of Entenmann's total packaged baked goods sold were these non-fat products.

I challenge you to find a better tasting coffee cake than their raspberry twist. Or a chocolate cookie that can match their chocolate chip brownie cookies. Or how about their non-fat carrot cake? And cinnamon rolls. Plus a wide variety of both yellow and chocolate cakes. With fudge icing. Yet these all contain absolutely no fat! We can eat all we want and it does not count at all against our day's allotment of saturated fat.

One of the many surprising things we discovered in developing the *Zap the Fat* program is that sugar has absolutely no bearing on our weight results. Unless there is a health reason for us to curtail our sugar, it need not be taken into account at all in counting what we consume each day. Since sugar contains no fat, it has no effect on our day's allotment of saturated fat.

When it comes to cooking things for breakfast, we can also use the same substitutes for eggs, butter, and oil, and come up with some very tasty and comforting dishes. This is even the case with waffles. Made the regular way they can check in with as many as 9 grams of saturated fat, even before the butter is poured on.

Here again manufactured products also can come to our rescue. Bisquick, for instance, is one of those who make a "light" mix that can be used to make pancakes with greatly reduced fat content.

Always remember to read the labels on those packaged products. For saturated fat content. For serving size. If it contains more than 1 gram in what would be a normal serving size, for us it is usually best avoided.

This can be particularly time consuming when we travel. We have gotten to know the facts on most of the grocery store foods we purchase and packaged products must show saturated fat and serving size on the box. But in a new area it can be quite different. Specialty breads, for instance, need to be checked for saturated fat. At home we have store-baked bran muffins that use egg whites and canola oil and are acceptable. But when we go to Massachusetts, the bran muffins have whole eggs and partially hydrogenated oils that are not acceptable.

CANDY

When it comes to candy it is very easy to separate our sheep from the goats. The culprit being saturated fat, all hard candies are always fine in any quantity. They contain none.

Unfortunately, very little chocolate candy can ever be all right for us. Candy bars, for example, average about 8 grams of saturated fat in just a single bar. Obviously they are not included in our eating plan.

Even something as seemingly innocuous as salt water taffy is usually a no-no. The reason: the ingredients include coconut oil. The same is the case with most packaged, already popped, popcorn. Remember, no palm, palm kernel, or coconut oil, since they are almost exclusively saturated fat.

The secret, then, with all candy, is to read the label. If it contains any butter, or anything with the word "butter" in it (e.g. cocoa butter), or any of the three forbidden oils, skip it. It is one of those things that we must learn to get along without.

When eating out, for instance, those candy striped hard mints often provided at the end of the meal are an excellent substitute for dessert. They give you the sugar kick without adding any grams of saturated fat.

For some of us it is very hard to re-program our thinking to realize that sugar is not the culprit. The culprit is the fat that is contained in many things that also contain sugar. But something made with sugar that does not also contain saturated fat does not need to be eliminated at all under *Zap the Fat*.

The bottom line on baked goods, desserts, and candies is then quite simple. All those listed in the No-Count Bread Products Table are fine in any quantity. Also, home-baked cakes, pies, and cookies made without saturated fat.

But there are many others which are not OK—commercially baked goods other than breads, rolls, bagels, and English muffins—desserts other than those that are made without the culprits of butter, whole milk, and oils—candies that contain any "butter" ingredient or one of the three bad tropical oils. We just can't include those in our *Zap the Fat* program.

If we are to meet and keep our correct weight goal, this is a decision we need to make. But with a little imagination and caution we can still feast on all the desserts and baked products we like, while avoiding the pitfalls of adding saturated fat to our diet.

WALLET CARD SUMMARY

BREADS, DESSERTS and CANDY

Count 0 grams SF—Bagels (without eggs), Bread, Bread Sticks (Plain), Buns (Hamburger or Hot Dog), English Muffins, Rolls (Hard, Soft, & French) - ALL Hard Candy

Count 1 gram SF—2 Graham Crackers, 6 Saltine Crackers, 2 Pancakes (4" diameter), Popover

Count 2 grams SF—Biscuit, Brownie, Chocolate Chip Cookie, Bran or Corn Muffin.

Count 3 grams SF—Cake Doughnut (no other type), Carrot Muffin, Cornbread

8

FROM SOUP TO NUTS (AND EVERYTHING ELSE)

A few food truths are as certain as death and taxes. One: any dairy product (unless it is NON-FAT) is going to contain saturated fat. Fact two: ditto for any type of meat. The third sure problem is nuts.

All nuts contain a lot of fat. Fat comprises at least 75% and up to 90% of the total calories in nuts. With the exception of brazil nuts, cashews, coconut, and macadamia nuts (which have twice as much as the others), all nuts contain almost exactly the same amount of saturated fat. (Chestnuts have none.)

A normal-sized portion (what you get in one of those little packages they give you on the airplane) is a half ounce (.5 ounce). It is easy to count the effect these have on our program, because the saturated fat in that half ounce portion of all the nuts we might eat—almonds, hazelnuts, peanuts, pecans, pistachios, sunflower seeds, and walnuts—always equals just 1 gram.

Because nuts are healthy in many other ways, I often choose to use them to consume some of my day's allotment when I am on an airplane. I'll eat a half ounce package of almonds or peanuts and count 1 gram of saturated fat for the day.

When traveling I am able to compensate for eating the nuts by ordering one of the low-fat meals that airlines offer all passengers who call 24 hours in advance to request it.

Unfortunately, two of my favorite nuts are cashews and macadamias. (Brazil nuts have never been one of my temptations.) However, as we see from the Nut Table, these three contain twice the amount of saturated fat found in the same-sized portion of other nuts—2 grams.

Consequently, part of my habit pattern reformation

NUT TABLE

(All reflect saturated fat in a .5 (one-half) ounce portion, unless otherwise noted.)

Item	Saturated Fat Grams
Chestnuts	0
Almonds	1
Hazelnuts	1
Peanuts	1
Pecans	1
Pistachios	1
Sunflower Seeds	1
Walnuts	1
Brazil Nuts	2
Cashew Nuts	2
Macadamia Nuts	2
Peanut Butter (2 tablespoons)	3
Coconut (3 tablespoons)	4

has been to decide that cashews and macadamia nuts can no longer be a part of my diet. Given the choice, I'd rather have twice the amount of almonds, or pecans, or even peanuts.

Another place I sometimes decide to splurge a part of my day's allotment is peanut butter. It contains 3 grams of saturated fat in two tablespoons. That is the amount on an average sandwich.

When I do take the plunge and go for peanut butter sandwiches for lunch, however, I make two of them. I use just one tablespoon of the gooey stuff on each one. With plenty of jelly or jam I end up with a very hearty lunch that still has consumed less than a third of my day's allotment of saturated fat. Not an unreasonable portion of my 10 grams to eat at lunch time.

One word of caution on peanut butter. Purchase the kind made without the addition of hydrogenated vegetable oils. Manufacturers add hydrogenated oils to make the product last longer out of the refrigerator. But those oils add more saturated fat to the peanut butter. Always check the label and get the kind made from nothing but peanuts and salt.

This is a good time to reiterate one of the primary pitfalls for those of us reading labels and trying to match them up with our personal *Zap the Fat* requirements.

Every label has two items that are imperative for us to take into account. One is the *saturated fat* in a serving. The other is the *size* of the *serving*. Under FDA regulations all packaged items must reveal both.

We need to ask ourselves whether the size serving shown on the label is the same size we expect to eat. If not, we need to do some further simple math.

For example, the serving size for peanut butter is always shown as two tablespoons. That adds three grams of saturated fat. But if I know I am not going to be happy without two sandwiches, and plan to put two tablespoons on each one of them instead of splitting it up between the two, then I need to face facts. I must double the amount of saturated fat I will get from that meal. Instead of 3 grams of saturated fat, I will get 6. In my opinion that is too much from one dish.

SOUPS

Soups are also items that will generally contain some saturated fat. The only exceptions are those that have been especially prepared without oil. That is always clearly specified on the label. Other exceptions would be those we make at home with no oils added.

The two main culprits in restaurant and homemade soups besides oil are creamed (milk) soups and the butter that a good chef often likes to add.

As a rule of thumb, assume that any canned creamed soup will contain 3 grams of saturated fat per one cup serving after addition of the required milk ingredient. Of course, if we use canned evaporated skimmed milk or regular skim milk instead, the saturated fat can be easily cut to half or even less.

For non-creamed soups such as chicken noodle, vegetable, and tomato, we need only assume we are getting a single gram of saturated fat in a normal one cup serving.

In addition, though, we must also watch what goes on our soup. Onion soup, for instance, is eliminated because of the saturated fat in the cheese that goes in or on top of it. Also, croutons have often been made with too much oil.

VEGETABLES and FRUIT

The saturated fat statistics regarding vegetables are simple and easy to remember. There are no vegetables that contain any saturated fat at all. There is absolutely no vegetable that we need to limit ourselves in eating. We can eat all we want without affecting our *Zap the Fat* program. Or our weight.

While all vegetables contain no saturated fat, the way we prepare them can, of course, do us in. For example, all those fried onion rings, fried zucchini, fried potatoes are out. Everything fried is just a no-no!

The same also applies to many ways potatoes are prepared besides being fried. Au gratin style includes cheese, and usually milk and butter, making them always a no-no. Even a 3-ounce sized portion (that deck of cards) of hashed brown potatoes contains 3 grams of saturated fat. If cooked in butter or bacon grease it will be even more.

My personal favorite has always been mashed potatoes. They are normally prepared with both milk and butter. However, I have found they are still quite good when skim milk is used and the butter is skipped altogether.

Fruits are almost as easy. There are just two fruits that, in their natural state, contain any saturated fat at all.

One of these is olives. However, in order to consume 1 gram of saturated fat you must consume 15 black olives, or several mouthfuls of 18 green olives. Consequently, even though olives do contain some saturated fat, we do not consider them in our counting, since the normal portion of a few olives will contribute negligible saturated fat.

The one fruit we do need to watch, however, is worth some serious attention. It is the avocado. A whole avocado contains 4 grams of saturated fat. If we put four thin slices on a salad or sandwich, that is about a quarter of a whole avocado. That will add 1 gram of saturated fat for those four slices. A half avocado will add 2 grams.

SNACKS

In addition to nuts, we also must also be wary of most snack foods. Obviously this would automatically include all that have been fried.

For example, there is a gram of saturated fat in 10 corn chips. Or 10 potato chips. And pray tell, who among us will limit ourselves to just 10 Fritos or Pringles? Even the so-called "reduced fat" or "low-fat" varieties still contain at least half the amount of saturated fat that is in the regular varieties.

The only exceptions in the chip field are those that have been baked instead of fried. Any amount of these will contribute nothing to our saturated fat allotment for the day.

The first manufacturer to enter the grocery market seriously with baked chips was Guiltless Gourmet. In addition to their line of chips they also have developed and marketed some excellent tasting bean dips (others usually contain lard), salsa, and even a fake nacho dip. All their products contain no saturated fat.

As more people get serious about eliminating saturated fat from their diets other manufacturers can be expected to join the baked chip bandwagon. Of course, we can also bake our own chips in the oven or microwave.

Popcorn is one snack that is great if we are careful. Regular microwave popcorn can contain as much as 2 grams of saturated fat in a regular 3 or 3 1/2 cup serving. Since I eat more than that at a sitting, the regular variety is out of the question for me.

However, there are very good tasting "light" varieties that contain only 1 or 2 grams of TOTAL fat, meaning their saturated fat is not countable. We can eat all of them we wish without cutting into our day's allotment. But we need to check the label to find those varieties containing "0" or "less than 1 gram" of saturated fat per serving.

Of course, we can also just air pop our own corn and accomplish the same purpose. By adding some spices we can give it even more flavor. Experiment!

That's it. We must choose wisely those items containing saturated fat which we decide to eat each day. Try to stick with foods containing just 1 or 2 grams in a serving the size we eat. And never let the total go over 10 grams for the day.

Eat to our heart's content. As much as we want of everything else.

There are so many interesting and good tasting foods out there. Once we learn the principle and develop the habit, we open up a whole new vista of eating pleasure without putting on undesired weight. Enjoy!

WALLET CARD SUMMARY

SOUP TO NUTS, etc.

NUTS *(per 1/2 ounce portion)*
Count 0 grams SF—Chestnuts
Count 1 gram SF—Almonds, Hazelnuts, Peanuts, Pecans, Pistachios, Sunflower Seeds, Walnuts
Count 2 grams SF—Brazils, Cashews, Macadamias
Count 3 grams SF—2 tablespoons of Peanut Butter

SOUPS *(per 8-ounce portion)*
Count 1 gram SF—non-creamed soups such as Chicken Noodle, Onion (without cheese or croutons), Minestrone, Tomato, Vegetable.
Count 3 grams SF—all creamed soups

VEGETABLES
Count 0 grams SF—Eat none prepared with butter or oils, or fried.

FRUITS
Count 0 grams SF—all EXCEPT olives and avocado
Count 1 gram SF—15 Olives
Count 2 grams SF—Half Avocado

SNACKS
Count 0 grams SF—Baked Chips (not fried), Popcorn without butter or oil, Pretzels

CONDIMENTS
Count 0 grams SF—ALL including Ketchup, Mustard, Red Cocktail Sauce, Salsa, etc.

9

MAKING EXERCISE SIMPLE

Exercise. Something to be avoided. Something I could never be any good at. Something reserved for the he-men (and women) of this world. Those were always my attitudes regarding exercise.

During grade and high school I was the youngest in my class. With an extremely small frame, yet tall for my age, I was also the least muscular of the group. Even as I grew taller I still could only be described as skinny.

I can remember the shame as I waited to be chosen for a ball team during recess. Always the last one. And the embarrassment during gym class when I found myself surrounded by a forest of strong, muscular legs.

It was small wonder that I conditioned myself to steer clear of all types of exercise. And particularly any that might require my appearance in all too revealing shorts!

Consequently, if a daily two mile walk had not been required by my doctors at Massachusetts General Hospital, I probably would have continued to resist exercise. Knowing what I do today, I realize that without that exercise *Zap the Fat* would not have worked so dramatically for me. Nor will it for anyone else who does not exercise.

Therefore, I want to share two simple forms of exercise. One is for the lower body and cardiovascular system, the other for the upper body. Both require a minimum of time, effort, and equipment. Both are easy to understand and do, and meet the *Zap the Fat* requirement for simplicity.

Before I start telling you about this simple program, however, I must give you the standard warning. Do not undertake this, or any exercise program, without first checking it out with your physician. Don't try any part of it unless you have his or her OK.

There is also a rule of thumb applied to our pulse rate that should always be followed to make sure we are getting as much exercise as we should, but also that we are not getting too much. To get that range:

• Subtract your age from 220—the resulting number is your maximum pulse rate.

• When you exercise your pulse should be at least 65% of that figure, but should never be more than 85% of it.

For example, let's assume you are 50 years old. Your maximum pulse rate would be 220 minus 50, or 170. 110 is 65% of that figure and should be your minimum pulse rate when exercising. 144 is 85% of that figure and that should be as high as your pulse rate goes when exercising.

THE WALK

It was with my negative attitude about exercise that I found myself leaving Massachusetts General Hospital in 1986 armed with some very firm instructions regarding the exercise I must undertake. Both my surgeon and my cardiologist told me that I must walk a minimum of two miles every day in a maximum of 30 minutes. That's at least 4 miles per hour.

If I did this, they assured me, I would be doing

everything possible for my cardiovascular system. No matter how much additional time I spent playing golf or tennis, or doing any other type of exercise, just spending those 30 minutes every day did all that could be done for the benefit of my heart and the cardiovascular system that supports it.

Since I had just spent over five weeks at their hospital recuperating from heart bypass surgery, I was ready to do almost anything to avoid a return engagement.

So I decided to give it a whirl. It took me about a month to get up to the necessary speed of a little more than 4 miles per hour. It works out for me to a pace of from 150 to 160 steps per minute.

After that first month I really didn't need to count any more. I found that I automatically walked at that pace whenever and wherever I started out on my morning walks.

In order to accomplish the two miles in under 30 minutes, however, I cannot ever stop during my walk.

A few months after I had started taking these daily walks, we took all of our children and grandchildren to a ranch in southern Arizona over Christmas.

One of my sons-in-law heard about my walking regimen and asked if he could come along one morning. I was delighted to have him join me.

About ten minutes into our walk in the desert we came upon a small herd of deer. "Look at that," he said, "let's stop for a minute and see what they do."

"Oh, no," I exclaimed, "if we stop now we'll have to start all over. We have to keep going."

So keep going we did. It was also the last time he has ever suggested he join me for a morning walk.

But if we had tried to divide the walk into a 10-minute and then a 20-minute period it would not have done the job on my cardiovascular system. It is the continuous 30-minute walk that causes the benefit.

In fact, I have found this is pretty much true of all my friends who think they might like to join me. Four miles an hour is a brisk pace. When you do it every day it doesn't seem so bad. But to a couch potato who wants to go out for a pleasant walk, it is definitely just too much.

I have another friend who prides himself on being in excellent shape. But he gets that way riding a bike. When he goes walking with me he ends up in a slow jog. His comment was that when they begin including "the scuttle" in the Olympics, he wants to enter me.

It just isn't a good social activity unless you have someone who is dedicated to doing it daily.

When I am in a strange city I am able to knock off my two miles in 30 minutes by walking one way for 15 minutes, then reversing my steps. At first I used a pedometer, but once my pace was set it was so inborn that I no longer needed one.

A word of caution: It is wise to keep very alert when walking in a strange city. I also ask a friend, or inquire at the hotel where I am staying, which is the safest direction to head out.

Once I was walking early in the morning in a park in Sydney, Australia. I heard voices coming toward me and looked up to see a half dozen rather threatening looking young men headed directly toward me. A quick turn at the rate of speed I was going led me away from them in very short order.

The same sort of caution has proven valuable in some quarters of Jerusalem. And in New York City. And, I must confess, these days just about anywhere. We must stay alert. Once our pace has become habit it is easy to center our concentration on our surroundings.

I do my walk every day and have done so for more

than seven years. When the weather is so bad I can't go outside I walk on a treadmill at 4.2 miles per hour. Most hotels today have an exercise room that includes a treadmill. I always inquire before making a reservation to ensure one will be available.

It doesn't make any difference where I am or what time of day, it is just part of my daily regimen. I do, however, find that going out when I first get up each morning keeps me on schedule and leaves little room for procrastination getting in the way later in the day.

THE WEIGHTS

Several years after I had begun walking, a close friend persuaded me that it would also help my overall health to take up simple weight lifting.

Because of my frequent travel, I told him I would try it on two conditions: that it be so simple I could do it anywhere, and that the weights I used not take up any extra room at home and be available when I was traveling at any hotel health club.

It is important again to insert a word of caution concerning lifting weights. When my blood pressure shot up at one point, my doctor told me to cease lifting weights until my blood pressure was brought back into bounds with medication. DO NOT BEGIN LIFTING WEIGHTS–OR WALKING–WITHOUT FIRST GETTING THE APPROVAL OF YOUR DOCTOR.

My friend took up the challenge and did it. He outlined a very simple six-step program that I now do three times a week. Never two days in a row. Always with at least one day of rest in between.

I use one set of regular 10-pound dumbbells. The entire daily program is all done lifting these two 10-pound weights, one in each hand, during each of the six different exercises.

Originally I was to do each exercise 10 times. Then, after a short rest (never more than one minute), to repeat the same group another 10 times.

After the first six months the schedule was increased to doing the two sets 15 times each, instead of just 10. I have never graduated above that level.

It is imperative that we keep our mouths open during these exercises. Also keep our knees slightly bent. And exhale (blow out) all the time we are exerting, which means every time we lift.

Here is a simple description of each of these six exercises that can be done using a set of 10-pound dumbbells. (For women the weight used can be less, as little as 5 pounds per weight. Find out what is comfortable for you at a gym.)

SQUAT *(Develops large muscles in front of legs)*

Set your feet apart. Both firmly on the ground. Hold one weight in each hand, arms loosely down to your sides. Bend your knees to a half squatting position with the bottom of your buttocks no lower than half way to your knees. Keep your back straight while doing this. Keep your heels on the floor. Return to upright position. Do it 10 times. Rest. Do it 10 more.

SHOULDER ROLL *(Develops muscles in upper back—also releases stress)*

Hold a weight in each hand. Arms at sides. Shoulders relaxed. Continue to hold the weights loosely to your sides. Rotate your shoulders (in the same way you would shrug them) easily from front to back, up and then back down. Repeat 10 times. Rest. Do it 10 more. Now reverse—rotate from back to front. Do that 10 times. Rest. Do it 10 more.

CURL *(Develops biceps)*

Hold a weight in each hand. Arms to sides, loosely. Lift both your hands to shoulder level. Keep your elbows close to your body. Your palms face to the rear as you reach shoulder level with the weights. Exhale as you do so. Then lower your arms back to the starting position at your sides. Repeat 10 times. Rest. Then do 10 more times.

MILITARY PRESS *(Develops triceps [back side of biceps])*

Hold a weight in each hand. Bend your arms, lifting the weights to shoulder level, elbows close to your body, palms facing forward, weights clenched in your fists. Now raise your arms above your head to their full length (palms continuing to face forward). Then lower the weights back to shoulder level. Repeat 10 times. Rest. Then do 10 more.

LAWN MOWER *(Develops large muscles of mid-back)*

Put weights on the ground on each side of you. Standing, face the seat of a chair or something of similar height. Bend your knees slightly and bend your body at the hip so that you are leaning forward. Place your left hand on the surface you are facing. Take a weight from the floor in your right hand. Keep your back parallel to the ground.

Brace yourself with your left hand on the chair and lift the weight in your right hand up to chest level, then return it to the ground. Lifting is done by bending your elbow and pointing it toward the ceiling. Don't move your body. Do this 10 times. Rest. Repeat 10 more times.

Now brace yourself on the chair seat with your right hand and take the other weight in your left hand. Repeat the exact same exercises with that hand. Repeat it 10 times. Rest. Do it 10 more.

CHEST PRESS *(Develops chest muscles)*

We get to lie on the floor for the last of our weight lifting exercises. Lie flat on your back. Take a weight in each hand and bring it up (any way it is easiest for you to do so) into the air, keeping your upper arms (from the shoulder to the elbow) flat on the ground, elbows close to the body.

Now lift the weights up, palms facing inward toward each other, to full arm length. Then lower them back to original position with upper arms still flat on floor, forearms perpendicular to the ground, and weights held in your hands. Repeat 10 times. Rest. Do it 10 more times.

That's it. That is your total *Zap the Fat* exercise program. Do a two mile walk in no more than 30 minutes. Do it every day.

Then do your weight lifting three times a week. While you should do your walk every day, it is equally important to always skip at least a day between your weight lifting.

That exercise is an imperative part of *Zap the Fat* was demonstrated by a condensation of an article from Forbes FYI in the February 1994, issue of *Readers Digest*.

A study by researchers Teresa A. Sharp and James O. Hill of the University of Colorado and their colleagues at Vanderbilt University showed that metabolism is the key to burning energy, and consequently weight loss. Their conclusion was that anyone can increase metabolism and weight loss by more activity: "stay moving."

They reported that "physical activity boosts metabolism by creating muscle and reducing fat." Yet Hill also reported it is not a short term thing but "it only works over the long term."*

If we expect *Zap the Fat* to work for us, regular exercise is a must. My wife can't walk long distances, but she is able to substitute for my daily walks with the same amount of time spent on a stationary bicycle. We all know that exercise plays an important part in keeping us healthy. It makes us feel better—and then feel glad we made the effort.

---

*From "The One (and Only) Secret to Permanent Weight Loss" by Terence Monmaney, *Readers Digest,* February 1994; condensed from "Thin & Now," *Forbes FYI,* September 27, 1993.

10

EASY EATING OUT (OR, HOW TO CONVERT YOUR FAVORITE RESTAURANT)

In my family eating out has always been a very special occasion. Even as a little kid I loved to dress up and go out to dinner with the family. It was a time of real celebration. I didn't even mind having to sit quietly and keep my voice down. It was worth it if it meant I could get dressed up and "eat out."

I remember when I was about eight years old my folks took me for the first time to the Sunday night buffet at the Kansas City Club. Just to be there in the oak-paneled dining room was a momentous occasion for me.

And that buffet! A lavish display of dozens of salads. Shrimp. Crab. Lobster. Smoked salmon. Five kinds of meat. Vegetables in all sorts of mouth-watering sauces. And desserts. Ah, the desserts. A veritable smorgasbord of rich cakes, pies, tortes—many of them goodies I had never even seen before.

After my heart surgery, when they began to talk to me in the hospital about limitations to be placed on what I could eat, I was crestfallen. Was I doomed to spend the rest of my life limited to a choice of whether I was going to take the vegetable plate or settle for a fruit platter?

Consequently, it was truly a new lease on life when my son, Philip, took pity on his poor father and began developing menu items at his restaurant that met the demands of my saturated fat regimen.

He demanded that those menu items not only be heart healthy but also taste good. Very good. He used the proper substitutes to make up for the missing fat. Flavor and taste were as much king as were the ingredient limitations.

When a balky landlord caused Philip to shut down his restaurant I was really depressed. Life had been so easy when I dined there. That had not been the case at most other restaurants.

For one thing I discovered that many restaurants all over the country marked various items on their menus with little hearts or other symbols. They claimed this identified heart healthy dishes.

But as my knowledge grew, I began to see that in most cases these symbols meant absolutely nothing. It was a gimmick with many restaurants. It was really worse than if they had staked no claims at all. At least in that case I could know I had to figure out for myself which food items were acceptable to my *Zap the Fat* limitations.

After his restaurant closed, Philip decided to translate his experience with the development of good tasting yet healthy eating alternatives into a new business. He set up a company called Heart Smart Restaurants International.

Heart Smart's purpose was, and still is, simple. It would help restaurants around the country develop, identify, and promote heart healthy menu items. With a trademarked seal of a heart with the word "smart" inside it, restaurants who bought into the Heart Smart program could provide the public with good tasting alternatives they could trust.

They set standards for an item to qualify for the Heart Smart identification: it must get 30% or less of calories from fat, 10% or less of its calories from saturated fat, contain 150 milligrams or less of cholesterol, and have no more than 1100 milligrams of salt. While only the saturated fat figure pertains to our *Zap the Fat* program, the 10% maximum pretty much guaranteed I could eat any qualified item and still stay on my program.

Every restaurant that becomes a Heart Smart client starts by getting its menu analyzed by the HSRI staff. They choose items that will probably meet the standards. The restaurant then sends in the recipes for those items.

A detailed analysis of the recipes is then made using the sophisticated Minnesota Nutrition Data System, the same system that Heart Smart used to provide all of the data on saturated fat you find in this book.*

Some of the recipes will already meet the Heart Smart standards. Others that may not qualify often can do so with certain changes. Cut the oil used in half. Use light mayonnaise instead of regular in a tuna sandwich. Substitute skim milk for whole milk. All of these are things we do when cooking at home as part of the *Zap the Fat* program.

The changes must not detract from the taste, however. This is, of course, important if the eating out experience is to remain an enjoyable social occasion. Just as it is important for us to keep the joy of eating with what we prepare at home.

Once Heart Smart has established the menu items,

---

*Heart Smart Restaurants International® performed all nutrient calculations using the Minnesota Nutrition Data System software, developed by the Nutrition Coordinating Center, University of Minnesota. Food Database version 7A; Nutrient Database version S22.

they also provide the restaurant with the Heart Smart Book, which lists the amount of fat, saturated fat, cholesterol, and salt in each qualified item.

Consequently, I am always able to find the grams of saturated fat in the item I am eating. Thus I know exactly how much I am adding to my 10-gram limit for the day.

Of course, in restaurants that are not part of Heart Smart, we still have to do our own calculating. But we still can eat well without bombing out on saturated fat. We just have to know what to ask. And be willing to stand up and do it.

If you're at all like me, this may be a problem. I am not a person who likes to be needy. Quite the contrary, I will go to great lengths to be the one who knows it all.

One time we dined at one of the most posh establishments in Phoenix to celebrate my birthday. Located in one of our many resort hotels, it had an excellent reputation. The ambiance was everything you could want. Lovely silver, crisp white tablecloths, crystal wine glasses. The food was also reputed to be beyond comparison.

Our waiter turned out to be just as impressed with himself as he was with the atmosphere in which he carried out his trade. At first I was sufficiently intimidated by my surroundings and his attitude that I considered forgetting all about saturated fat for the evening. After all, it was my birthday.

But then I saw that old self-deception for what it was and decided to get needy. I explained to him the first time he came around to our table, while his attention was riveted on the drink order, that I had to limit the saturated fat I ate. Therefore I had a few questions about the menu.

"Nonsense," he retorted, "this is not McDonalds.

QUESTIONS FOR RESTAURANTS

Cooking Ingredients

• Will they cook everything I order without using any butter or animal fats?

• Will they use canola oil or olive oil for anything which requires oil?

• Will they advise me if there is cheese on anything I am ordering? Often there is cheese when it is not mentioned on the menu.

• Will they use skim milk or other non-fat dairy products whenever they use any dairy in preparation?

Cooking Method

• Will my meal be prepared using one of our acceptable methods of preparation? (Baked. Broiled. Grilled. Poached. Roasted. Steamed. Stewed. Sauted in wine, its own juices, or something else besides butter or oil.)

• Will they give me the portion size I desire? I want a meat portion to be from three to a maximum of six ounces. No more or I'd go over my day's allotment.

• Will they remove the skin from poultry?

• Will they remove all visible fat from other meat before cooking it?

Serving Method

• Will they serve my sauces and dressings on the side? This applies to salads, main dishes, even some vegetables. (Seeing the amount of the dressing I am putting on a salad is, of course, the only way I can control how much saturated fat I am consuming.)

• Will they refrain from adding anything to my vegetables, such as a glob of butter just before it leaves the kitchen?

• Will the waitperson work with me to solve my needs and help make this meal a memorable occasion?

Everything here is loaded with fat and butter. That's what makes it good."

This is where I had to give up and really bite the bullet. I realized my attitude was not reflecting my very real need. Granted, looking up at his nose held high in the air didn't make it easy. But what were my priorities? To get the best of this waiter and put him in his place? Or to get a good tasting, low saturated fat meal?

"I'm sorry," I replied, "but I really am serious about what I eat. I must limit my intake of saturated fat, and I do need your help and that of your chef if we are going to do that."

And miracles of miracles. The nose came down. The satisfaction of being legitimately needed lit up his face. He became my friend and confidant. He joined forces with me. He took my requests to the chef and saw that they were honored. He ended up with a satisfied customer and a good tip.

Once I really made up my mind that I was going to be open and needy in any restaurant I visit, I began to discover some very specific things I could do to make every meal a pleasant, yet healthy, experience. I just must know what I need and ask the waitperson to help me.

There is a small restaurant we frequent in the little town of Cornville, Arizona, where we live. The chef, Albert Kramer, was trained in Switzerland and has been in the restaurant business for more than 40 years. His whole family before him was as well.

Because of a heart problem, he left the rat race in California, where he had a very successful restaurant, and came to our little Arizona town. He also got serious regarding the saturated fat in what he cooked.

We frequently eat at his restaurant as do many people, some of whom drive two hours up from Phoenix just to savor his special dishes. And they are good.

Yet he cooks everything with canola oil. Many dishes are done just in a reduction of their own juices with all the fat skimmed off.

He even has four desserts that contain no saturated fat at all—including a flan covered with caramelized maple syrup, another called Chocolate Velvet, a rich, creamy dish that is the first cousin to a chocolate mousse.

I can go into his Manzanita Inn and eat like a king without any regrets the next morning. Sometimes more than once a week. He is living proof that it can be done. All we have to do is educate the staff in the restaurants we frequent about how to do it. As bearers of the *Zap the Fat* message, we can easily do that.

It is even easy to follow *Zap the Fat* when visiting our favorite fast food restaurants. Many of them, such as Boston Chicken (which had all its menu items analyzed by Heart Smart Restaurants International) and McDonalds, show the saturated fat content along with other data on posters prominently displayed on the wall at each of their restaurant locations or on printed handouts available for the asking.

You must keep up to date with these posters and handouts, however. For example, until early 1994 McDonalds offered a low-fat chocolate milk shake with just 1 gram of saturated fat. I was going to recommend it in these pages. But then they changed the recipe and their charts today show they now make it with 4 grams of saturated fat, way too much for our program.

We already know from our *Zap the Fat* Wallet Card the saturated fat content in a card deck-sized piece of broiled chicken without skin. Consequently, we can still easily handle eating out at fast food chains even if they have not provided the statistics.

We also need not be discouraged by ethnic restaurants. For instance, let's take Mexican. Heart Smart has

PLAN OF ACTION FOR RESTAURANT EATING

1. Make the decision you are going to be needy. Swallow your pride and be ready to let your waitperson know you are serious about what you are going to put in your mouth. And expect cooperation. Don't let yourself be intimidated by an uninterested attendant.

2. After you are seated, study the menu. Eliminate all the known no-no's like fried items, creamed items, fatty meats. From the others choose a couple that appeal to you and question your waitperson about them.

3. Get more needy.

4. Ask the waitperson to remove butter from the table unless there are others with you who eat it. Never let them put any on your butter plate.

5. Ask for sauces and salad dressing to be served on the side.

6. Question cooking ingredients as well as methods using your knowledge of what is acceptable. Be specific about fat-laden foods that are not to be used (butter, milk products other than non-fat, cheese, whole eggs, etc.).

7. For dessert choose fruit or sorbet unless the restaurant has some non-fat specialties (e.g. many restaurants now offer non-fat frozen yogurt for dessert).

a chain of 27 Mexican restaurants as clients. Their menu includes more than two dozen different items that qualify as being Heart Smart. Their refried beans, for example, contain no fat, saturated or otherwise. A flour tortilla spread with them tastes as good as those using regular lard laden refried beans.

Even when I visit a Mexican restaurant that doesn't take healthy eating seriously, however, I can still do so. Instead of gobbling up those fried chips, for instance, I order three warm flour tortillas without butter. They are every bit as good when dipped into the nice hot salsa. Then I ask the waiter how they prepare the items that might be acceptable and choose those that can be made properly.

We have a friend who has a large, black purse. It always accompanies her when eating in a Mexican restaurant. When the time comes, she opens it to reveal her stash of non-fat sour cream and grated non-fat Alpine Lace yellow cheese. The dishes have been ordered with no sour cream or cheese, of course. But dressed up with the contents from her purse they suddenly perk up to look like their saturated fat-loaded compatriots at other tables.

The same applies to Italian fare. We need to avoid any white or cream type sauces. Instead, we can eat all we want of marinara (red) sauces that contain no meat. Or, if I am willing to use some of my day's allotment, I can choose a garlic and olive oil spaghetti sauce.

In all of it, of course, we come back to the question: have we made the decision? Once we have made up our own minds, the rest is easy!

We first develop the new habit pattern in our home consumption and cooking methods in order to *Zap the Fat*. Then, if we want to have the same success when we eat out, we must continue with that same decision. Once that is done, all we need to do is follow our predetermined Plan of Action (see previous box).

Statistics show that Americans spend about half their dining dollars eating away from home. That's a lot.

Since I travel a lot, I eat out often. If I were to let down my guard and decide to follow the path of least resistance when I do, it would soon be reflected in my weight and my health.

But I do value the celebration aspect of a good meal in a fine restaurant. Maybe if enough of us insist on that as a right to which we expect to be entitled, we will begin to find increasingly large numbers of restaurants who do as much for us as Albert does in Cornville, Arizona, and the restaurants who have joined Heart Smart Restaurants International.

11

IF CHOLESTEROL AND/OR SODIUM ARE YOUR PROBLEM

(Counting cholesterol and sodium is NOT a part of the Zap the Fat *program. However, many who follow* Zap the Fat *do so to lower cholesterol and/or blood pressure. Consequently, the following simple plan to deal with cholesterol and sodium is included for them.)*

My father had some interesting eating habits. Today they would be considered shocking.

Every day his lunch consisted of a ham and swiss cheese sandwich, loaded with mayonnaise. For dessert he would top it off with a piece of coconut cream pie. If by chance they were out of that, he would settle for banana cream. And often a chocolate milk shake.

Then, every night before he went to bed he indulged in a large dish of strawberry or chocolate ice cream.

He was always in a hurry. We used to say he always ran. I don't think I ever saw him walk. He seemed to have very little weight problem, except for an abundance around the waist.

That continued until at the age of 61 he had a debilitating stroke. It paralyzed the left side of his body for the remaining 13 years of his life.

Until this point everything we have been looking at pertained to the saturated fat content of the foods we eat. Our sole emphasis has been on reaching our proper weight and maintaining it for the rest of our lives.

Some of us with family histories like mine, however, have problems caused by what we eat that go beyond weight. One of these is a high cholesterol level that can lead to heart disease and strokes. These are at least partly caused by both the cholesterol and the saturated fat in the food we eat.

Sodium is another cause. For some people—it's estimated about 30% of us—excess sodium consumption contributes to high blood pressure (hypertension), a major factor in strokes.

CHOLESTEROL

As previously mentioned, I started the *Zap the Fat* program because of my own problems with high cholesterol and heart disease. In addition to its effect on them, I discovered quite by accident that cutting down saturated fat in my diet to 10 grams a day also eliminated excess pounds and brought me down to my normal weight. And continuing the *Zap the Fat* program meant that I maintained my proper weight regardless of what else—or how much of it—I ate.

Cholesterol has only come to be recognized for the culprit it is during the last generation. However, I realize my family history reveals that high cholesterol levels have obviously been a major problem over the past several generations.

Besides my father, my paternal grandfather and grandmother, as well as my maternal grandfather, suffered debilitating strokes in their 60s. It didn't take much gray matter for me to realize there had to be something in my genes that warranted attention to cholesterol.

We now know our cholesterol levels should run under 200. When they are between 200 and 230 they are considered "borderline." Over that is getting dangerously high.

Prior to the time of my heart surgery, my cholesterol had hovered in the area of 325 to 350. About six months before the surgery, my doctor had tried a drug to bring it down. That particular drug left my liver all screwed up, and was identified by my doctors at Massachusetts General Hospital as being what caused me to develop pancreatitis while recovering from the bypass surgery.

I was really rather indignant, since most people get pancreatitis from long over-consumption of alcohol. But though I didn't abuse alcohol, mine behaved exactly the same. The doctors told me that my pancreatic enzymes were eating away on my liver and stomach. There is no known cure.

The only treatment is to stop eating or drinking anything (including water) until the pancreas decides to return to normal and stop its overproduction. Not too many years earlier, this disease usually proved fatal. However, they had developed a new method of handling the situation. It saved my life.

They inserted a long needle into my mammary vein. They fed me 1800 calories a day through it. An ominous looking bottle containing a yellowish liquid was placed on the stand by my bed regularly at two o'clock every afternoon. For the next 24 hours it dripped all the food and liquid I needed into my body through my chest.

For five weeks I neither ate nor drank anything by mouth. I got up religiously four times a day to take my walk down the hall. Everyone got to know me. The man pulling the stand on rollers with the yellow bottle hanging on it. The rollers were old and often stuck in the wrong position. But everywhere I went it had to accompany me. Even to the bathroom.

Consequently, after all that I didn't need anything more to motivate me. I was willing to do everything possible to control my cholesterol.

Previously, I had half-heartedly tried to eliminate many items from my diet that contained cholesterol. But obviously with little success, since my count was still way over 300.

So I began to get serious about understanding just what it is that causes high cholesterol. The most surprising thing I discovered was that the actual cholesterol in the foods I ate was not the primary culprit. Rather, it was the saturated fat in what I ate that caused my liver to manufacture more cholesterol than it needed. In fact, the cholesterol that my consumption of saturated fat stimulated my liver to manufacture was twice the problem of that created by the cholesterol I actually consumed.

The University of California *Wellness Letter* states that cutting down on saturated fats "is the most important dietary step you can take" to reduce cholesterol levels. They point out that a high intake of saturated fats not only raises total cholesterol but also increases the so-called "bad" kind: LDL, low density lipoproteins.

This means that those of us who seriously adopt the *Zap the Fat* program benefit from a byproduct to our weight loss and control. We have also taken the single most important step we can to reduce our cholesterol as well. The program even helps raise the "good" cholesterol: HDL, high density lipoproteins.

The *Wellness Letter* reports that another major factor involved in increasing HDL and decreasing total cholesterol is the loss of weight. Indeed, it states that "not only does excess body fat raise your total blood cholesterol and LDL and reduce HDL, but it also appears to be an independent risk factor for heart disease."*

*Excerpted from the University of California at Berkeley *Wellness Letter*, December, 1993. ©Health Letter Associates, 1993.

So, by seriously embarking on the *Zap the Fat* program we have already taken two giant steps toward cholesterol control. There remains just one other main factor: actually reducing the amount of cholesterol we ingest from the food we eat. Most doctors recommend a reduction to 150 milligrams of dietary cholesterol a day.

We have been able to simplify the identification of foods that contain that old devil saturated fat. We did this with a method by which we can count to 10 and limit ourselves to a daily maximum allotment of saturated fat. It is possible to watch our daily cholesterol consumption using an equally simple formula.

First, it is encouraging to know that we already have eliminated most cholesterol-containing products by following the *Zap the Fat* program. Take milk, for instance. Skimmed or non-fat milk, the only kind we use, contains only a few milligrams of cholesterol in an 8-ounce glass. We don't even need to count this against our daily limit of 150 milligrams.

The same applies to any dairy product. If it is identified as "non-fat" in content then we do not need to count it as providing any cholesterol. No cholesterol to be counted. No saturated fat to be counted. This applies to all dairy products that are non-fat—cheeses, milk, ice cream and yogurt, etc.

The same is the case with butter in baked goods. Butter is a real menace because it adds cholesterol to our diet, just as it adds so much saturated fat. We have already eliminated it entirely. Margarine, on the other hand, although it contains some saturated fat, contains no cholesterol at all.

The only foods we do need to consider that are allowable under the *Zap the Fat* saturated fat guidelines are meat and eggs. Other than these, everything else that could be a problem already has been eliminated.

There are just two items in these categories that are totally unacceptable:

- Egg yolks, which contain about 250 milligrams of cholesterol in each yolk (there is absolutely no cholesterol in the whites—see Chapter 4)
- Organ meats, which can contain several hundred milligrams of cholesterol depending on the particular organ meat you eat. Eliminate such things as liver, kidney, brains, etc. No great loss if you're anything like me.

It is evident that eating either egg yolks or any organ meat will put us way over our maximum 150 milligrams of cholesterol for a day. So we need to forget they exist if we are watching our cholesterol.

Since everything else containing cholesterol has already been eliminated, meat is the only other food we need to consider. Regardless of what kind of meat it is (except organ meat)—whether fish, chicken, red meat, whatever kind—we always count each one ounce portion of that meat as containing 25 milligrams of cholesterol. That's all there is to it. (There is one exception: shrimp. It runs about 45 milligrams per ounce.)

Actually, the exact amount of cholesterol per ounce does vary with the type of meat. But that variance is slight—some are as low as 20, others as high as 30. But by using our simple 25 milligrams per ounce quotient, we will average out correctly. And it is easy to count.

In Chapter 5 we explained how our saturated fat alert leads us to count 3-ounce portions of fish, chicken, and meat. That is the portion shown on your Wallet Card. That is the portion we always use as a measure. You'll recall it is a portion the size of a deck of cards.

Consequently, whatever 3-ounce portion we eat of any type of meat should be counted as 75 milligrams of cholesterol. If we eat two such portions a day, we have consumed our 150 milligram maximum. It is that simple.

If we don't eat meat on a given day, we may assume that we have consumed no cholesterol. But remember this is on the assumption that we have followed the rest of the *Zap the Fat* program. If we cheated and ate regular milk products or butter, for example, we would have consumed considerable cholesterol. In addition to the saturated fat they contained.

There are many things we can eat instead of meat, of course. Vegetables, salads, pasta (with red sauce or olive oil—no cream sauce unless made with skim milk), grains and breads of all sorts, and fruit. None of these contain any cholesterol at all.

The object of our personal cholesterol count is to get it below 200. For someone with my problems, a combination of the *Zap the Fat* program, limiting cholesterol intake to 150 milligrams a day, exercising, and taking a drug to keep it low brings mine down to about 225. While with my genes that is a miracle, most people who limit their cholesterol consumption to no more than 150 milligrams a day will easily find their cholesterol count drops below 200 without drugs and stays there.

SODIUM

For a number of years I followed the *Zap the Fat* program with my attention riveted on just saturated fat and cholesterol intake. My tests showed that all was well.

Then one day my doctor announced that my blood pressure was up to 165 over 95. Thus began a new part of my journey into food realities.

Normal blood pressure is supposed to be 120 over 80. Still, they usually don't get concerned if the lower figure (diastolic) stays under 90, and as long as the upper one (systolic) stays under 160.

My doctor told me that they used not to be concerned with a systolic reading unless it exceeded your age plus 100. If I'd just been born 20 years earlier I would have appeared normal! (Of course, if I'd been born 20 years earlier I probably wouldn't have lived to anywhere near my 60s without benefit of a debilitating stroke.)

But studies over the last 10 years have shown that there is now more concern when you have a systolic pressure reading higher than 140 (as a risk for stroke and heart attacks) than with a slightly elevated diastolic reading. I was definitely "at risk" and needed to do something about my blood pressure. Now!

Part of my problem, I knew, was stress. I am very adept at manufacturing my own if ever there is not enough around me.

The Bible says people my age are supposed to sit in the gates of the city. To dole out wisdom. Not to try to run everything. Or really almost anything. To be available where we're needed. But not to run around trying to sniff out ways to make ourselves needed. To get out of the rat race as much as possible.

So my doctor and I agreed that control of my stress should help reduce the blood pressure. But the other culprit that needed my attention was salt.

He told me to limit my salt intake to 3,000 grams a day. Some doctors want it as low as 2,400. In extreme cases, even less. As with saturated fat and cholesterol, I realized that if I was to do that I needed to have a simple formula I could follow easily.

I concluded that by eliminating from my diet foods which contained more than 400 grams of sodium, the daily total should never exceed my 3,000 gram limit.

I discovered that there are certain types of foods that consistently exceed 400 grams in a portion. By eliminating all of them would I succeed in keeping my total consumption under 3,000?

For example, almost all fresh fruits, vegetables, meats, and breads fall way under the 400 limit. I don't need to pay any attention to them at all. I can eat all I want.

On the other hand, there are a few things that I have had to eliminate altogether, even though they were acceptable in the saturated fat and cholesterol areas.

ITEMS TO BE ELIMINATED ALTOGETHER FOR SALT CONTROL

PROCESSED OR CANNED FOODS—Unless the label clearly shows there are less than 400 grams of sodium in a portion (and the portion is the size I will really be eating), all processed or canned foods are out. If the label doesn't show the sodium at all then I must assume it is over 400 and can't use it.

The exceptions to this are canned vegetables and fruits which are identified as "no sodium," "low sodium," or "1/2 the sodium." These are OK.

It is estimated that fully a third of all the sodium we consume comes from processed foods. Manufacturers use it to help preserve their canned goods since it helps inhibit the growth of the bacteria that cause things to spoil.

SOUPS—This was a hard one for me. I probed for a way to get around it. There just isn't one.

Whether canned or bought in a restaurant, any soup is going to contain way over 400 grams of sodium. In fact, you should assume any of them contain at least 700 grams, and more often than not it will be over 1,000.

Soups are just not something we can have unless

they are homemade and we know no salt has been added. The only exception is canned soup showing on the label that it contains under 400 milligrams of salt per serving.

TOMATO JUICE and TOMATO BASED PRODUCTS— This hurts. One of the joys of *Zap the Fat* is that you can still have all you want of so many good things made with tomatoes. Chili with the right quantity and type of meat in it. Spaghetti sauce. Barbecue Sauce.

But if you also need to watch your sodium you must be careful of any of these that come out of a can. Or is served in a restaurant.

For example, a glass of tomato juice runs from 900 to 1,000 grams of sodium.

Again, of course, if you make them yourself from scratch, you can eliminate the sodium. Unfortunately, you won't find tomato juice without salt that has much taste.

Other no-no's are: cottage cheese, olives and pickles, soy sauce, Worcestershire sauce, etc.

In addition to these that must be eliminated, some others also need to be watched. While they may contain less than our 400 figure "per serving," they can add a lot of sodium with a little quantity.

For instance, a tablespoon of mustard adds 200 grams. A tablespoon of ketchup about 150. An English muffin can run up to 350 grams. A regular muffin about 200. Even though none of them will add to our saturated fat, it is just wise to be aware of this when we must be careful of our sodium intake.

About a third of the sodium we get in our diets comes from salt added to food in cooking or at the table. Obviously, the first and easiest step I took was to eliminate that salt shaker at the table. We have cooked without added salt for years as a general health measure. The only salt shaker we have in the house sits on the top shelf of a kitchen cabinet and is reserved for guests who demand it.

When we make anything from scratch we can cut way down on the sodium. In fact, if we didn't use canned things, including soups and tomato products, we could control the sodium very easily.

There are a lot of good ways to make up for the salt. Lemon juice is probably the best known flavoring agent for use as a salt substitute.

Other substitutes include:

Basil

Chives (also freeze-dried)

Dry Mustard

Fruit Juices

Garlic (and Garlic Powder)

Ginger

Horseradish

Hot Sauces (may contain salt but a little goes a long way)

Marjoram

Mrs. Dash and other salt-free granulated products

Onion (and Onion Powder)

Oregano

Parsley

Pepper

Sage

Sun-Dried Tomatoes

Thyme

Vinegar

The cholesterol and sodium facts, then, come down to another very few, easy to follow, instructions.

First, follow the saturated fat limits and eliminate the items outlined as part of the *Zap the Fat* program.

If, like me, you need to lower your cholesterol, also eat no more than 6 ounces of fish, meat or chicken a day. And eliminate egg yolks and organ meats.

If you need to limit your sodium as well, also eliminate canned or restaurant soups, other canned foods, canned tomato products, cottage cheese, olives, pickles, and soy sauce. The only exception would be those canned products that state on the label that they contain under 400 grams of sodium per serving.

12

POSTSCRIPT

Corrie ten Boom was a fascinating lady who died back in the 1980's. During the Second World War, she spent several long years in a German concentration camp. Her parents and her sister all died there. Yet she maintained a strong faith in God and great simplicity of character through it all.

After the war, she came to the United States and began to share her faith and wartime experiences in churches throughout the country. Her words and books inspired hundreds of thousands of people, and she helped many who had borne grudges for years to come into the joy of granting real forgiveness. Just as she had learned to do with her guards and captors.

In the midst of all this fame, just as she had done in the midst of her suffering in the concentration camp, she often repeated an admonition to her audience: KISS. Translated: KEEP IT SIMPLE, STUPID!

I like to think of KISS as the motto for the *Zap the Fat* program. As we've already seen, it is definitely not a diet program. In fact, we only use the word "diet" as a noun in this book, used to describe what we eat. It is never used as a verb, to describe something we do.

Zap the Fat has to do with just that: what we eat. We have tried to keep it all in very simple terms. KISS! This holds true whether we are talking about counting the 10 grams of saturated fat we eat every day. Or the cholesterol we consume. Or the salt in our food. Or the way we exercise.

I know from my own battles there is no way any plan can work for me if it isn't kept simple. At the same time, I know the only hope for my own health and well being is to have settled the saturated fat issue for the rest of my life. Period!

You can buy books with countless pages of tables including decimals to show the exact amount of fat and saturated fat in each item. To make *Zap the Fat* simple, we instead round off each decimal to the nearest whole number. Even when you do this with a column of hundreds of numbers, the result will come out within one of what it would have been if the decimals had been used. Thus we accomplish the same result while keeping it very simple and easy to use.

If we can count to 10, and can add figures that total 10, we can succeed at the *Zap the Fat* program. It is really pretty difficult to get very haughty about a major change in lifestyle that is this simple.

But as we have also discovered, adopting the *Zap the Fat* life-style change is just like giving up smoking. We must make a decision to do battle for a season with a lifetime of bad habits. But once we have made that decision, and taken that step, all the results which follow will bring us more peace. More victory.

I have a good friend who had a major heart attack followed immediately by the same heart bypass surgery I had experienced a few years earlier. Frequently, we eat lunch together along with several other men. It's one of those "bring your own lunch" affairs, held in one home or another.

In the first few months after his heart attack and

surgery, his wife was very cautious in what she prepared for his lunch. He would sometimes ask me for advice on how he could spice up the taste of one item, or whether there was any saturated fat in another. He was really enthusiastic about the program, and he prospered with it.

After those first few months, however, I noticed his lunches began to take on a different hue. Potato chips were sneaking back in from time to time. The cream cheese in his sandwich, he told me, was "light" but not "non-fat." "After all," he said, "I don't fix my own meals. I just eat what my wife puts on my plate."

Then one evening I was at their house when his wife was preparing their dinner. I noticed her putting a large dollop of butter on top of the vegetables. "Blanche," I moaned, "you're not really going to put butter on the vegetables for Bud to eat, are you?"

There was fire in her eyes as she replied: "I'm just not a fanatic like you, John! After all, Bud isn't dying."

I was really saddened. Because as long as that life-time decision had not been made, it meant that Bud *was* dying.

As another friend of mine says, eating is a lot like gravity. Its effect on your weight won't change no matter how much you pray. Our rebellion pulls us steadily back into the overweight corner, until we decide it's not worth staying there.

Just as with a person who joins Alcoholics Anonymous (AA), the only way to claim the victory is to take it one day at a time. The AA member has made a decision to give up drinking for life. Looking ahead, that seems an impossible undertaking to him. Consequently, even though he has made the lifetime decision, he knows this decision must be worked through just one day at a time.

Even after years of success, that same AA member can suddenly fall off the wagon. After sobering up, he takes a look at what pressures caused the fall. Then seeks forgiveness and turns back with his face to the sun to live out this lifetime decision–again one day at a time.

Those of us who make the *Zap the Fat* decision are exactly like the AA member. We may fall off the wagon. Usually it will happen when we are out to dinner or visiting friends. We don't want to go through the hassle or the embarrassment of letting our needs be known.

Or we may just decide to rebel and eat a whole fried chicken. Or a large order of french fried onion rings. Or a double chocolate cheese cake. Or a big bag of potato chips.

In fact, a survey reported in *Parade* magazine showed that 46% of the respondents in 1992 said that they were binging from time to time. This compared with just 36% who made the same claim a year earlier.

The times I have fallen off the wagon I have found it very important to ask a friend to help me see what triggered my disdain for what I know is right for me and what I genuinely embrace as a way of life. Then I can repent of the cause.

Right away, I count up the total grams of saturated fat I ate during my binge. That whole fried chicken, for instance, would come in at about 30 grams. Each of the onion rings at two grams. The cheese cake at 22 grams. The bag of potato chips at a gram for each 10 chips— depending on the size of the sack, from 6 to 20 grams of saturated fat.

I find it very important to know just how much I have overeaten. Then I make a conscious effort to hold the next few days' totals at a level which, when averaged with my binge totals, still will come out at just 10 grams. It may take a week, or even longer, but recovery is possible no matter how bad the binge. The secret is to count the cost of that binge as soon afterward as possible. And to take the necessary action at once.

We also need to make the decision to reverse the lies that have become a part of our lives, and govern so much of our behavior. I have one friend, a marvelous cook, who was excited about *Zap the Fat*. She raved to me about how great it was, "except I must, of course, use a little butter now and then." With this basic attitude she had already lost her battle.

If we are to truly succeed at zapping the fat for the rest of our lives, that word "except" just can't be a part of our vocabularies. That applies to whole milk products (including butter), fried foods, organ meat or meat fat, and almost all commercially baked products.

I had been told since I was a small child that eating liver was necessary for good health. That almost nothing tasted good unless it was made with butter. That what makes vegetables great is adding plenty of salt pork or bacon. That no Sunday dinner was complete without plenty of fried chicken. And breakfast had only one definition: bacon and eggs!

But I have had to accept the fact that every one of these supposed truths is in reality an outright lie. I find the only way to reprogram myself against those lies is to pray and ask the Lord to forgive me for believing each lie as it comes up, and then to ask him to reprogram me and set me free from believing that lie. It works! Just like we would reprogram a computer, He can reprogram what makes us tick.

We are overwhelmed with data that proves we need to change our eating habits. The World Health Organization reports that in 1900 the United States was the #1 healthiest country in the world. Today it ranks #93. They say this is entirely because of our diet.

A study by the National Cancer Institute found that non-smoking women who ate diets with 15% or more saturated fat were six times more likely to develop lung cancer than those with diets containing 10% or less. By following the *Zap the Fat* program with its 10 gram per day limit, we are consuming only about 5% of our diet in saturated fat.

Another study done by Dr. Edward Giovannucci, instructor of medicine at Harvard Medical School in Boston, was quoted in the publication *Health Confidential*. It reflected data from a study of 48,000 men. The study found that those who ate the most red meat, butter, and chicken with skin (things eliminated or included only in great moderation with *Zap the Fat*) were two and a half times more likely to develop late-stage prostate cancer than men who ate the least of these foods.

These are just two of the plethora of studies that show the relationship between saturated fat consumption and heart disease, many types of cancer, and other diseases.

Doctors tell us we actually need no saturated fat at all in our diet. (We do need some other types of fat.) The body will manufacture all of the saturated variety we need.

So a decision to follow *Zap the Fat* is a total win/win situation. It causes us to lose weight and find and retain our proper weight for the rest of our lives. And it practically guarantees that our lives will be healthier and more likely to be free of major illnesses such as heart disease and cancer.

We need to see that *Zap the Fat* differs in many ways from diets. It does not count calories. One reason for this is that a gram of fat contains more than twice the calories in a gram of carbohydrate. But the main reason is that counting calories is just too complicated.

Zap the Fat is also in no way affected by sugar. We can eat all we like. There is no saturated fat in sugar.

In fact, we can eat most foods as explained on the *Zap the Fat* Wallet Card. Using that card, we can limit ourselves to no more than the specified count of 10 grams of saturated fat per day.

It is possible to cheat the system if we were determined to do so. For example, if we used up all 10 of our saturated fat grams one day by eating 10 tablespoons of canola oil we would end up consuming way too much overall fat. But if we are eating normally, the percentage that comes from canola oil will be offset by that which comes from meats wherein a much higher percentage of the fat is saturated.

What works best for me is to consume no saturated fat grams for breakfast. I also avoid any snacks during the day that contain saturated fat. I just eat those listed on the *Zap the Fat* Wallet Card.

Normally, I limit myself to no more than 3 grams at lunch. That leaves me 7 grams for dinner. Very often there are days when I never reach the total of 10 this way.

When eating foods that do include some saturated fat, I try to limit myself to those which have just 1 gram, or at most 2. Very occasionally I may go for a 3. These are all shown on the *Zap the Fat* Wallet Card.

We live in a world of options. Such a life has spawned hundreds if not thousands of diets over the years.

My mother was one of those who spent her life trying different diets. She was the one who introduced me to the diet with all the eggs. Just five feet tall herself, she fought a constant battle with her weight. Her weapon was whatever new fad diet was popular at the moment.

Yet she was never happy with the results. She was a

permanent rider on the merry-go-round. And she died of cancer at the age of 60.

Julia Childs is recognized as one of the foremost chefs in the world. When she talks, everyone listens. She was quoted as saying, "I get very depressed if I don't eat well." Her method of cooking, however, seems to continue endorsing cooking with butter and ignoring the saturated fat problem.

Graham Kerr is another of the world's famous chefs. He knows the importance of eating well and feeling you ate well after you have done so.

When his wife, Trina, suffered a stroke some years ago he did a major study and came to the conclusion that fat was the culprit. Since then he has devoted his life, and his TV programs, to showing us how we can eliminate the saturated fat in classic dishes and still retain all their pleasure-giving, good tasting quality.

Despite all the options open to us, everything comes back to just one thing: cut way back on the saturated fat in our diet and we will:

- lose weight permanently and keep it off
- feel better
- look better
- avoid much of the risk of heart disease and cancer

NO DIET can offer us all of these benefits. But the *Zap the Fat* combination of low saturated fat eating and simple yet consistent exercise does so for life.

Trivia: The number of Americans trying to avoid dietary fat in 1993 dropped by 4% from the number ten years earlier in 1983. This according to a study done by American Health Habits, Baxter International, Deerfield, Illinois.

We can only assume that people have become discouraged trying to deal with counting the 40, 50, or

even 60 grams of fat that they eat every day. The sim-
plified solution of counting just 10 grams of saturated
fat can overcome that resistance.

If we are ready to get honest with ourselves—to take
a step and break the habit patterns of a lifetime for the
rest of our days—to give up the suicidal track of the diet
carousel—my experience indicates that we can be blessed
beyond our wildest dreams.

Is it worth it?

APPENDIX 1

DESSERTS THAT MAKE IT ALL WORTH WHILE

A good friend of mine has spent more than 25 years in the diet business. She has helped thousands of suffering dieters to face the problems in their lives that make their weight bounce up and down like a yo-yo.

Because of her experience, she was one of the first to whom I exposed the *Zap the Fat* program. She was very excited.

And I was excited that she was excited. Until she started talking about all the "excepts." She just couldn't comprehend something that was permanent. For life. Without any "excepts."

Most particularly she was concerned about entertaining. "There are just certain recipes I always use when I am entertaining. What would they be without butter? Or cheese? And bacon? And what would dessert be without Mrs. McElhenney's Tennessee Frozen Fudge Cake?"

That seemed bad enough until we got on the subject of fried foods. She has some marvelous little deep fat fried hors d'oeuvres that delight many of her guests. "I think I can probably stay away from fried things 85% of the time," she explained. With a straight face!

I was really frustrated. How is anyone going to permanently *Zap the Fat* by eliminating fried foods and Tennessee Frozen Fudge Cake just 85% of the time? Or by insisting that those other specialties of so many years are the only acceptable dishes to serve when entertaining? Obviously she wasn't!

Then the light dawned. The permanent dieters really seem to enjoy the roller coaster ride. They rationalize as "reality" the fact they will diet a while. Go back to things the way they have always been. Gain some weight back. Diet a while again. Ad nauseam.

That conversation persuaded me something needed to be included in this book to let the permanent dieter realize there is hope. That you don't have to use saturated fat to make things taste good.

Originally I had not wanted to include any recipes. There are so many good sources of such recipes, including magazines like *Cooking Light*. But what about a few really gummy, gooey, dessert recipes that include no more than 1 gram of saturated fat per serving? Some even rich in chocolate. Would that help everyone realize there is hope after *Zap the Fat* for delicious eating?

My wife was born and brought up in the South. She always says, "forget French pastries and anything whipped. I like my desserts real sweet and gummy." If these recipes satisfy my wife, believe me they will take care of anybody's sweet tooth.

Therefore, here are the recipes. They are ones that we and our friends have developed and shared with one another. The saturated fat per serving is shown at the bottom of each recipe. They are all delicious. Guaranteed to satisfy our sweet tooth. To give us hope that everything is to be gained except undesired weight when we get serious about *Zap the Fat.*

SORBET

Serves 25

1 1/2 cup sugar
1 1/2 cup water
1 cup fresh mint leaves
1 16 oz can crushed pineapple
3 lemons, squeezed
3 oranges, squeezed
3 bananas, mashed
3 egg whites

Mix sugar, water and mint in a saucepan. Bring to boil and simmer 1 hour. Let cool and strain. In bowl mix the pineapple, the orange and lemon juices and the mashed bananas. In large beater bowl whip the egg whites to stiff peaks. Carefully fold in the pineapple-juice mixture and the mint flavored sugar-water. Place in ice cream freezer and freeze according to freezer directions.

Count 0 grams saturated fat per serving

APPLE CRISP

Serves 9

5 to 6 cups peeled, cored, thinly sliced cooking apples
3/4 cup quick-cooking rolled oats
3/4 cup brown sugar
1/2 cup all-purpose flour
1 tsp. cinnamon
1/3 cup canola oil

Arrange apples in greased 8x8-inch pan. Combine oats, sugar, flour, cinnamon and oil. Sprinkle mixture over apples. Bake at 350° for 35 to 40 minutes or until apples are done. Serve warm with whipped dessert topping (see recipe) or frozen non-fat yogurt.

Count 1 gram saturated fat per serving

PRUNE SOUFFLE OR WHIP

Serves 4

1 cup strained cooked prunes
3 egg whites
1/3 cup sugar
1/4 tsp. salt
1 Tbl. lemon juice
1/4 cup chopped walnuts

Heat oven to 350°. Beat prunes, egg whites, sugar and salt until stiff. Fold in lemon juice and walnuts. Pour into ungreased 1 1/2 quart casserole. Place in larger pan of very hot water (1-inch deep). Bake 30 to 35 minutes or until puffed and thin film has formed on top. Serve warm with whipped dessert topping (see recipe).

Count 0 grams saturated fat per serving

BAKED CUSTARD

Serves 6

3/4 cup egg substitute
1/3 cup sugar
1/4 tsp. salt
1 tsp. vanilla
2 1/2 cups skim milk, heated
Nutmeg

Heat oven to 300°. Blend egg substitute, sugar, salt and vanilla. Gradually stir in hot milk. Pour into six, 6-ounce custard cups. Sprinkle with nutmeg. Place cups in baking pan, 13x9 inches. Place pan with custard cups on oven rack; then pour very hot water into pan to within 1/2 inch of tops of cups.

Bake about 45-60 minutes or until knife inserted halfway between center and edge comes out clean. Remove cups from water. Serve custard warm or chilled.

Count 0 grams saturated fat per serving

CARAMEL CUSTARD   Serves 6

Before preparing Baked Custard recipe (without the nutmeg), heat 1/2 cup sugar in small heavy pan over low heat, stirring constantly, until sugar melts and is golden brown. Divide syrup among custard cups. Allow syrup to harden about 10 minutes.

Pour custard mixture over syrup. Bake. Invert custard cups to unmold and serve warm, or chill and unmold at serving time.

Count 0 grams saturated fat per serving

BREAD PUDDING   Serves 20

8 slices bread
3/4 cup chopped walnuts (optional)
3/4 cup raisins

Crumble bread into oiled 9x13 pan. Sprinkle nuts and raisins over the bread and mix in a little.

1/2 cup sugar
1/2 tsp. salt
   Mix together and add:
3/4 cup + 2 Tbl. egg substitute
2 tsp. vanilla
6 cups non-fat milk
   Mix and pour over crumbled bread
1 tsp. cinnamon
1 tsp. nutmeg
   Sprinkle over top.

Set pan in larger pan with about 1/2 inch hot water. Bake at 325° for approximately 1 hour or until knife comes out clean. Cut into 4"x5" pieces.

Count 0 grams saturated fat per serving

CHOCOLATE BREAD PUDDING
Serves 20

Make Bread Pudding recipe but
Add to sugar:
1/4 cup extra sugar
1/2 cup cocoa
Blend together well before adding liquid ingredients.

(Raisins and nuts may be omitted)

Count 1 gram saturated fat per serving
Count 0 grams saturated fat per serving if walnuts eliminated

HOT FUDGE PUDDING CAKE
Serves 9

1 cup flour
2/3 cup sugar
1/4 cup cocoa
2 tsp. baking powder

1/4 tsp. salt
1/2 cup skim milk
2 Tbl. canola oil
1 cup chopped walnuts

Measure flour, sugar, cocoa, baking powder and salt into a bowl. Blend in skim milk and oil. Stir in nuts. Pour into ungreased 8x8 inch pan.

2/3 cup brown sugar
1/4 cup cocoa
1 3/4 cup hot water

Stir together brown sugar and cocoa. Sprinkle over batter. Pour hot water over batter. Bake 350° for 20-25 minutes. Should be runny on bottom. Serve quite warm, inverting each piece onto plate and spooning sauce over top. Serve topped with non-fat vanilla yogurt.

Count 1 gram saturated fat per serving

TRIFLE
Serves 8

1 Entenmann's Non-fat Pound Cake
1/2 cup raspberry preserves
1/3 to 1/2 cup dry sherry (or fruit juice)
1 16 oz can peach slices (Lite) (or apricot halves)

1 small package Jello brand vanilla pudding mix
3 cups non-fat milk
1 tsp. vanilla extract
1/2 tsp. almond extract
1/4 cup slivered almonds, toasted (optional)
1/2 cup non-fat whipped topping

Cook the pudding according to package directions, using the 3 cups of skim milk. Stir in the extracts.

Slice cake into 1/2 inch slices. Place half the cake slices in the bottom of a pretty glass serving bowl. Sprinkle with half the sherry or fruit juice. Spread half the raspberry preserves on the cake. Place half the peach slices (apricot halves) on top.

While pudding is still hot, pour half over the cake slices. Repeat the layers as above. Cover and chill thoroughly. Before serving garnish with Whipped Dessert Topping and toasted almonds.

Count 0 gram saturated fat per serving

BLACK FOREST CHEESECAKE   Serves 12

Filling:
3/4 cup graham crackers, crushed
2 (12-ounce) packages fat-free cream cheese product,
softened
1 1/2 cups sugar
3/4 cup egg substitute
1/2 cup unsweetened cocoa
1 1/2 tsp. vanilla extract
1 (8-ounce) carton non-fat sour cream alternative

Spread graham cracker crumbs on bottom of a 9-inch
springform pan coated with cooking spray. Set aside.

Beat cream cheese product at high speed with an
electric mixer until fluffy. Gradually add sugar, beating
well. Gradually add egg substitute, mixing well. Add
cocoa and vanilla, mixing until blended. Stir in sour
cream alternative. Pour into pan.

Bake at 300° for 1 hour and 20 minutes. Remove from
oven; run a knife around edge of pan to release sides,
but do not remove cake from pan. Let cool on wire rack.
Cover and chill at least 8 hours.

Topping:
1 (21-ounce) can reduced-calorie cherry pie filling
Whipped dessert topping (see recipe)

Remove sides of pan, and spread with cherry pie filling.
Dollop each serving with whipped dessert topping (see
recipe).

Count 0 grams saturated fat per serving

CHOCOLATE-AMARETTO CHEESECAKE or CHOCOLATE-MINT CHEESECAKE

Make filling as for Black Forest Cheese Cake adding:

2 Tbl. all-purpose flour
1/4 cup Amaretto or Creme de Menthe
Bake as directed
Serve with dollop of whipped dessert topping (see recipe)

Count 0 grams saturated fat per serving

CHOCOLATE MARVELS   Yield: 4 dozen

1 tsp. instant coffee granules
1 tsp. hot water
3 egg whites
1/2 tsp. vanilla extract
3 cups sifted powdered sugar
2/3 cup cocoa
2 Tbl. flour
1/8 tsp. salt
1 cup chopped walnuts

Dissolve coffee granules in hot water in a bowl. Stir in egg whites and vanilla. Combine powdered sugar, cocoa, flour and salt in a beater bowl. Add egg white mixture and beat at medium speed with an electric mixer until blended. Stir in nuts. Drop by rounded teaspoonfuls 1-inch apart onto greased and floured cookie sheets. Bake at 350° for 12 to 15 minutes. Remove to wire racks to cool.

Count 0 grams saturated fat per serving

CHOCOLATE TORTE   Serves 12

1/2 cup canola oil	1/2 cup water
1 1/2 cups sugar	2 cups all-purpose flour
2 egg whites	1 tsp. baking soda
1/4 cup egg substitute	1/4 tsp. salt
1 cup non-fat buttermilk	1/2 cup cocoa

Beat together oil and sugar. Add egg whites, one at a time, beating after each addition. Add egg substitute and beat. Combine buttermilk and water. Combine dry ingredients; add to sugar mixture alternately with butter-milk mixture, beginning and ending with flour mixture. Blend well, but do not overbeat.

Pour batter into two 8-inch round cake pans coated with cooking spray. Bake at 350° for 20-25 minutes or until a toothpick comes out clean. Cool in pans on wire rack 10 minutes; remove from pans and let cool completely.

FROSTING for CHOCOLATE TORTE:

1/3 cup cocoa	1 cup non-fat milk
1/2 cup sugar	1/4 tsp. vanilla extract
1/4 cup cornstarch	

Combine thoroughly the cocoa, sugar and cornstarch in the top of a double boiler. Stir in non-fat milk. Bring water to a boil. Reduce heat to low; cook, stirring con-stantly with a wire whisk, 18 minutes or until spreading consistency. Stir in vanilla. Cover and chill.

3/4 cup no-sugar-added raspberry spread
Fresh raspberries (optional)
Fresh mint sprigs (optional)

To assemble cake: stir raspberry spread well. Slice each cake layer in half horizontally. Place one layer on plate;

(continued)

spread with 1/4 cup raspberry spread. Place cake layer on top and repeat procedure with next two layers; top with fourth layer.

Spread frosting on top and sides of cake. If desired, garnish with raspberries and mint sprigs.

Count 1 gram saturated fat per serving

CHOCOLATE FUDGE CAKE   Serves 9

Cream together: 1 cup sugar
                1/3 cup canola oil
                2 egg whites
Sift together: 1 1/4 cups flour
                1/3 cup cocoa
                1 tsp. baking soda
                1 tsp. salt
Add: 1/2 cup non-fat buttermilk
                (or 1/2 cup non-fat milk with 1 Tbl.
                vinegar)
                1/2 cup boiling water
                1 tsp. vanilla

Combine first two mixtures and add liquid. Pour into 8x8-inch pan which has been sprayed with cooking spray and bake at 350° 25-30 minutes or until done.

FUDGE FROSTING:
1/4 cup water   1/2 tsp. vanilla
1/3 cup cocoa   2 cups powdered sugar

Heat water. Blend cocoa and sugar. Add slowly to water and beat, adding vanilla, until of spreading consistency.

Count 1 gram saturated fat per serving

WHIPPED DESSERT TOPPING

Almost freeze a suitable amount of evaporated skim milk, then whip it. (You get a very large amount when it is whipped; since it cannot be stored successfully, make only enough for the amount to be served.) One quarter cup will serve 4 to 6. Put the milk in the freezer in a bowl large enough to be used for beating. When milk is almost frozen, beat at high speed, adding one or a combination of the following:

sugar or sugar substitute to taste
almond or vanilla extract
brandy or cognac
cinnamon or nutmeg
instant coffee granules
cocoa

Count 0 grams saturated fat per serving

CHOCOLATE SAUCE

About 2 cups sauce
Serves 8

1/2 cup cocoa
3/4 cup sugar
2/3 cup evaporated skim milk
1/3 cup light corn syrup
1 tsp. vanilla

Combine cocoa and sugar in saucepan; blend in evaporated milk and corn syrup. Cook over medium heat, stirring constantly, until mixture boils; boil and stir 1 minute. Remove from heat; stir in vanilla. Serve warm over non-fat ice cream, non-fat frozen yogurt, etc.

Count 0 grams saturated fat per serving

HOT FUDGE SAUCE

Makes about 3 cups sauce
Serves 12

1 can (14 1/2 ounces) evaporated skim milk
2 cups sugar
3/4 cup cocoa
1 tsp. vanilla
1/4 tsp. salt

Thoroughly combine sugar and cocoa in heavy sauce-pan. Add evaporated skim milk and bring to rolling boil, stirring constantly. Boil and stir for 1 minute and 15 seconds. Remove from heat and stir in vanilla and salt. Serve warm.

Count 0 grams saturated fat per serving

CHOCOLATE BOSTON CREAM PIE

Serves 12

6 Tbl. cocoa
6 Tbl. sifted cake flour
1 cup plus 2 Tbl. granulated sugar (keep separate)
1/8 tsp. salt
8 large egg whites
1 tsp. cream of tartar
1 tsp. vanilla extract

Preheat oven to 375°. Line bottoms of two 8-inch round layer cake pans with wax paper.

Sift together cocoa, flour, 1 cup sugar and salt. Set aside.

In the large bowl of an electric mixer, beat egg whites at moderate speed until foamy. Add cream of tartar and remaining 2 Tbl. sugar, 1 at a time. Beat until soft peaks hold. Increase the speed to moderately high, add vanilla extract and beat 1 minute longer. The whites should be soft and firm, not stiff and dry.

(continued)

With rubber spatula, gently fold the cocoa mixture into the egg whites, about 1/3 at a time, then carefully pour the batter into the cake pans.

Bake 20 to 25 minutes or until they begin to pull away from the sides of the pan and a toothpick inserted in the centers comes out clean. Remove and cool on a wire rack upside down in the pans. When cool, loosen sides, turn them out and remove wax paper.

FILLING for BOSTON CREAM PIE:

1 cup skim milk	Pinch of salt
2 Tbl. all-purpose flour	1/4 cup egg substitute
2 Tbl. sugar	1/2 tsp. vanilla extract

Heat milk in heavy saucepan. In mixing bowl combine flour, sugar and salt. Stir some of the milk into the flour mixture, combining well, then pour mixture back into saucepan. Cook on medium heat stirring constantly until it thickens and boils, about 1 minute. Pour some of the pudding mixture into the egg substitute. Combine well, return it to saucepan as before and cook briefly, stirring constantly. Remove from heat; stir in vanilla extract. Cover and set aside to cool.

FUDGE FROSTING for BOSTON CREAM PIE:

1 cup sugar	1/8 tsp. salt
1 Tbl. white Karo syrup	3 Tbl. cocoa
1/3 cup skim milk	1/2 tsp. vanilla

Mix sugar, Karo syrup, skim milk, salt and cocoa. Cook in a heavy saucepan over low heat to soft-ball stage, or 238°. Remove from heat, add vanilla, and beat until cool. To assemble cake, place one cake layer on serving plate, spread with filling. Top with second cake layer. Spread frosting on top, letting it run over the edge of the cake a little.

Count 0 grams saturated fat

APPENDIX 2

UNDERSTANDING PACKAGE LABELS

Today the Food and Drug Administration requires that all packaged products clearly show certain nutritional information on their labels.

Only two of the statistics shown are of interest to us in our *Zap the Fat* program:

**Serving Size
and
Saturated Fat**

Shown here is the **Nutrition Facts** label from a brand of cereal that I frequently eat. You will note it shows the following information:

Serving Size: 1 cup
Saturated Fat: .5 g

Since I normally eat 1/2 cup of this cereal, and not a full cup, my saturated fat intake would be 1/2 the amount listed.

Nutrition Facts

Serving Size 1 cup (56 g)
Servings Per Container about 8

Amount Per Serving

	Cereal Alone	with 1/2 Cup Vit A&D Fortified Skim Milk
Calories	220	260
Calories from Fat	25	25
		%Daily Value**
Total Fat 3g*	5%	5%
Saturated Fat 0.5g	2%	2%
Polyunsaturated Fat 0.5 g		
Monounsaturated Fat 1g		
Cholesterol 0mg	0%	0%
Sodium 260mg	11%	14%
Potassium 230mg	7%	12%
Total Carbohydrate 44g	15%	17%
Other Carbohydrate 30g		
Dietary Fiber 4g	17%	17%
Sugars 9g		
Protein 7g		

Consequently, I am getting only .25 grams (1/4 of a gram) of saturated fat from my regular morning bowl of cereal with skim milk. In the *Zap the Fat* program, saturated fat UNDER .5 grams (1/2 of a gram) is not counted at all, and .5 grams (1/2 of a gram) and above is counted as a full gram. Therefore, my cereal consumed does not count at all.

By noting the serving size and the saturated fat grams on any packaged food, we can quickly tell what that will add to our daily allotment of 10 grams of saturated fat.

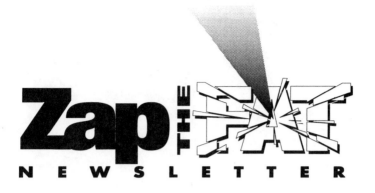

NEWSLETTER

If you are interested in receiving a free sample copy of the *Zap the Fat* Newsletter, fill in the form below and return to: **Paraclete Press**, Southern Eagle Cartway, Brewster, MA 02631 or call **1-800-451-5006.**

☑ **YES! I would like to receive a free sample of the Zap the Fat Newsletter!**

Name _____

Street _____

City _____

State _____ Zip _____

Phone ( ) _____

ZAP THE FAT
WALLET CARD

Following is your *Zap the Fat* Wallet Card. It is the simple key to success in following the *Zap the Fat* program.

The card shows the grams of saturated fat found in items that are all right to eat. These items have been divided into categories in the same order they appear in chapters 4-8 of this book.

In those chapters, we showed the grams of saturated fat for all foods. Even those which are much too high to be included as part of our healthy eating program.

On the card, we have listed the foods that contain up to 2 grams of saturated fat per serving. In a few cases we have also listed those with 3 grams. None any higher.

We have not included brand name foods you buy in the supermarket. They all show the amount of saturated fat and serving size on their packages. Consequently, you purchase them based on the information found on the package. It is not necessary to show them on the card.

You MAY eat as much as you like of anything containing 0 grams of saturated fat. You may also eat other things packaged or listed on the card where there are 1, 2, or sometimes as much as 3 grams of saturated fat. Providing, of course, you eat the serving size that is shown to contain that amount. And don't exceed a total of 10 grams per day.

On the card we use the abbreviation SF to mean Saturated Fat. We use gr as the abbreviation for grams. Therefore SFgr means grams of saturated fat.

Remove your wallet card, fold it, and put it in your wallet. You already know how to count to 10 so now you have all you need to embrace the *Zap the Fat* eating habit.

Errata

In Chapter 11, all references to <u>grams</u> of sodium should read <u>milligrams</u>. For instance, on page 114, it should read: " . . . limit my salt intake to 3,000 <u>milli</u>grams a day."